HORMONE BALANCE

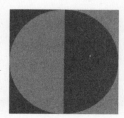

A WOMAN'S

GUIDE to

RESTORING

HEALTH and

VITALITY

CAROLYN DEAN, M.D., N.D.

Adams Media
Avon, Massachusetts

*To my sisters by birth and my sisters by choice and my sisters
who don't yet know how connected we are one to another.*

Published by
Adams Media, an F+W Publications Company
57 Littlefield Street, Avon, MA 02322. U.S.A.
www.adamsmedia.com

ISBN: 1-59337-333-3

Printed in Canada.

J I H G F E D C B A

Library of Congress Cataloging-in-Publication Data
Dean, Carolyn.
Hormone balance / Carolyn Dean.
p.   cm.
Includes bibliographical references and index.
ISBN 1-59337-333-3
1. Endocrine gynecology—Popular works. 2. Women—Health and hygiene—Popular
works. 3. Reproductive health—Popular works. 4. Hormone therapy—Popular works.
5. Hormones—Popular works. I. Title.

RG159.D426 2005
618.1—dc22
2005009560

This publication is designed to provide accurate and authoritative information with regard
to the subject matter covered. It is sold with the understanding that the publisher is not
engaged in rendering legal, accounting, or other professional advice. If legal advice or other
expert assistance is required, the services of a competent professional person should be
sought.
—From a *Declaration of Principles* jointly adopted by a Committee of the
American Bar Association and a Committee of Publishers and Associations

Many of the designations used by manufacturers and sellers to distinguish their product are
claimed as trademarks. Where those designations appear in this book and Adams Media was
aware of a trademark claim, the designations have been printed with initial capital letters.

Hormone Balance is intended as a reference volume only, not as a medical manual. In light of
the complex, individual, and specific nature of health problems, this book is not intended to
replace professional medical advice. The ideas, procedures, and suggestions in this book are
intended to supplement, not replace, the advice of a trained medical professional. Consult
your physician before adopting the suggestions in this book, as well as about any condition
that may require diagnosis or medical attention. The author and publisher disclaim any
liability arising directly or indirectly from the use of this book.

*This book is available at quantity discounts for bulk purchases.
For information, please call 1-800-872-5627.*

Contents

Acknowledgments

I WOULD LIKE TO THANK AND ACKNOWLEDGE the editors at Adams Media for asking me to write a book on women's hormonal health, not knowing that it was a secret dream of mine. I thank my agent, Jacky Sach, who thought I could pull off the impossible for Adams when they needed a writer to produce an already scheduled *Everything*® *Alzheimer's Book* within six weeks. Always one to rise to the challenge, I managed both to deliver the book and keep my sanity! Immediately after that adventure, Adams asked me to write *Hormone Balance*. I was thrilled. It has been a joy to research and write this book, which I hope will touch the lives of many women and their loved ones.

Hormonal wellness is but one of the many stages of wellness in women's lives. My twenty-five years in the medical field began with the desire to give people, and mostly women, tools to achieve optimal wellness. *Hormone Balance* is a milestone in my journey of service.

I would like to further acknowledge the journey that I have been on and the amazing people who have helped me to bring wellness to women for the past several decades.

First are the thousands of women in my former private practice in Toronto, who gave me the blessed gift of their confidence as we walked a path of wellness together. These were and are women awakening to their inner voices urging them to grow in body, mind, and spirit. I was privileged to share their journey. I learned from these women that when two or more people are united in the same experience, the journey is halved.

Slowly, my focus on medicine took an unexpected path. After thirteen years of private practice, my patients were evenly divided between people who wanted to focus on wellness and preventive medicine and people who were very ill and for whom I was the last resort. Because of the latter group I was persuaded to move to New York and research a medical modality that could treat chronic fatigue syndrome, fibromyalgia, and HIV. After many years that modality evolved, with the help of a remarkable woman, Delia Quigley, into the Body Rejuvenation Cleanse (BRC). The BRC diet along with organic herbal tinctures is designed to help detoxify the body from the environmental, infectious, physical, and emotional stresses that block our path to wellness.

During the formative years of BRC, I also worked with another wonderful woman, whom I mentored when she was a medical resident in 1985. Dr. Margaret Merrifield and I always knew we would work together in some capacity. Around 1995, we began brainstorming about how to teach wellness and how to convey the wellness concept to the general public. By 2004, Dr. Merrifield, in her clinic in Richland, Washington, had created a health care system that she felt doctors could implement in their practices.

However, I still wanted to work with the public. Hosting Body Rejuvenation Cleanse workshops, I soon learned that not all people are ready for such a monumental change in their lifestyle. For participants to be successful in the BRC program, they had to come with an established level of commitment to make the necessary changes in order to become healthier. For example, in Manhattan, Delia and I were challenged by people who had never cooked a meal; who stored their shoes in their oven; and who thought sugar was a food group!

A further challenge came for me when I tried to work with a women's business group to increase their health awareness. I reasoned that, since women are responsible for most of the health care decisions and health care buying in the family, businesswomen would be the group that could learn about wellness and then lead their families and their employees toward better health.

In January 2004, I had an opportunity to give a health seminar to a group of high-powered and high-pressured businesswomen at a spa retreat in Puerto Rico. It was disappointing. To begin with, most of the women opted to relax on the beach instead of being lectured to about what was wrong with their lives. Who could blame them? And of the women who were present, the only tendril of advice they said they "might" be able to implement was to *drink more water*! For the most part, these women's lives were too overwhelming to add one more thing to the dozens of balls they were already juggling in the air.

At this point, I was really at a loss because I knew I wanted to help women get healthy and stay healthy. I knew from my experience in private practice that you start with the first step and each successive step is easier because the enormous benefits of increased energy and well-being kick in. But I didn't have a vehicle. My dilemma was soon answered. Because the world works in wonderful ways, as a result of that spa retreat, I met another amazing woman.

Elizabeth Crook is a life and business coach for groups and individuals. She enthusiastically supports ethical investing and responsible business practices that nurture the individual, the local community, and the globe. She is also the daughter of Dr. William Crook who I had met back in the mid-1980s. Dr. Crook wrote *The Yeast Connection* and many other books describing the intrusion of Candida albicans into our lives. Candida is a yeast that overgrows when women take the birth control pill, antibiotics, eat too much sugar, and lead stressful lives! Yes, most of us are affected!

In the 1980s, I was treating yeast in my practice; was an advisor to the Candida Research Foundation of Canada; and ended up on an Ontario television show with Dr. Crook in 1986. It was a ninety-minute call-in show that clocked about 80,000 calls, which was a record for that show. A letter from the producer also said that the station's phone lines were jammed for days afterward and the mailroom was backed up with requests for transcripts.

Dr. Crook passed away in 2002 and Elizabeth took over her father's company to continue to provide his books and his key insights to women. She asked me to be advisor to a newly formed Women's

Health Connection and its joint Web sites, *www.yeastconnecction.com* and *www.womenshealthconnection.com*. In a beautiful full circle, I was reconnected to my work with yeast and with women, in general.

The next piece of the puzzle was solved by Jim Strohecker who has pioneered the Internet adaptation of Dr. John Travis's Wellness Inventory. If you came to know *Hormone Balance* through the Women's Health Connection, then you are aware of the Women's Wellness Inventory that we have developed from the Wellness Inventory. If you do not know of the Women's Wellness Inventory, you are in for a treat. The Women's Wellness Inventory gently probes twelve areas of our lives giving hints and clues as to the areas that might need your attention.

1. Self responsibility and Love
2. Breathing
3. Sensing
4. Eating
5. Moving
6. Feeling
7. Thinking
8. Playing and Working
9. Communicating
10. Sex
11. Finding Meaning
12. Transcending

Happiness with your answers is indicated on a separate satisfaction score. If you are dissatisfied with where you find yourself in any of these twelve areas of living, Women's Health Connection provides resources to help you reach your goal. Each step of the way, it is your choice to proceed further. Most diet books and health books fail because someone else is telling you what to do. Even if you think the premise is sound and you go along with it for the first few chapters, at a certain point you say to yourself "forget it." Nobody likes being told what to do. That's why the Women's Wellness Inventory begins with self-responsibility and love. Nobody else can be responsible for your health and when you learn to love yourself you have the confidence to start your journey. I invite you to acknowledge your own wellness and come on the journey of wellness that I have begun at *www.womenswellness inventory.com*.

Introduction

PUBERTY IS ARRIVING YEARS before it should, the birth control pill (BCP) is being given to twelve-year-olds, and many women are infertile by the age of thirty. What are the connections among these facts? And what does a decade or more of using the pill, followed by a few years of taking fertility drugs, do to the delicate balance of female hormones? Millions of women baby boomers are trying to understand where—and if—hormone replacement therapy (HRT) fits into their lives. Today, more and more women are searching for safer ways to balance their hormones.

Hormones are measured in tiny amounts called nanograms and picograms. Depending on the stage in your menstrual cycle, normal levels of estradiol for a woman can fluctuate from 50pg/ml to 300pg/ml. How small are these amounts? Consider the following:

- One milligram = one-thousandth of a gram
- One microgram = one-millionth of a gram
- One nanogram = one-billionth of a gram
- One picogram = one-trillionth of a gram

Once you know that a nanogram is one billionth (1 with 9 zeros) and a picogram is one *trillionth* of a gram (1 with 12 zeros), you can get an idea of the power of hormones and better understand how our hormones can so easily be thrown out of balance.

HRT has been used since the 1950s. It was in 1966 that Dr. Robert A. Wilson was commissioned by the makers of Premarin to sell a nation of women on the age-defying benefits of an estrogen substitute derived from pregnant mare's urine. In the forty years since then, we have begun to learn more about the side effects of HRT. Over that same time period, the chemical xenoestrogens in our environment that mimic hormones have been jamming up hormonal receptor sites in a process that Dr. Candace B. Pert (in her book *Molecules of Emotion*) calls "chemical rape."

Hormone Balance describes the incredible orchestration of hormones in the body and the many ways that balance can be disrupted. This loss of balance can lead to symptoms of mood swings, PMS, weight gain—and even seizures. Hormones (or her-moans, as my sister Chris calls them) are definitely something that women moan about, and there are a multitude of reasons why. In this book, I hope to give you a better understanding of your hormones, let you know why they may be out of balance, and provide you with numerous ways to achieve hormone balance and harmony within yourself.

In *Hormone Balance*, you'll find that the choice you face is not just whether to take HRT or whether to tough it out. There are many more ways that you can be involved in taking care of your hormones. These include diet; exercise; herbal, vitamin, and mineral supplements; and bioidentical HRT. With the right information and support, you can make your menopausal years happy and healthy.

In 1999, I wrote a small book on menopause called *Menopause Naturally*. Even though that was only a few short years ago, I'm amazed at the incredible amount of information and research on female hormones that has sprouted since then—both medical research and volumes of information on the Internet. It is both exciting and overwhelming. Unfortunately, much of the Internet information you encounter is associated with companies trying to sell their products, so is inherently biased. To help you sort through this maze, in this book I'll be analyzing the most up-to-date research, and translating often-complicated medical and technical knowledge into workable solutions.

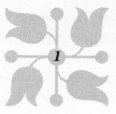

Who's Suffering Now?

WHAT DOES IDEAL hormone balance look like in the twenty-first century? Let's begin by describing that ideal, and then we can compare it to what's really happening with our hormones. In North America today, the norm is that most young women go on the BCP and stay on it for decades; infertility is reaching epidemic proportions; perimenopause has been labeled a new hormonal disease; and most menopausal women have to choose between HRT and its side effects or menopausal symptoms.

The Ideal Life Cycle

Naturally, the life cycle begins with the sperm and the ovum (egg). By extension, the health of this union depends on the health of the owners of the egg and sperm. Ideally, both partners would abstain from cigarettes, alcohol, coffee, over-the-counter drugs, and prescription medications for the six months prior to conception. They would eat organic food that was free of genetic engineering, pesticides, herbicides, hormones, and the other chemical adulterants common in factory-farmed and processed foods. For both partners, stress would be at a minimum, as it would be regulated by prayer and meditation, deep breathing, daily exercise, and a loving and grateful attitude toward life and other people. Yes, this may sound impossible for you and me, but let's just continue.

A Peaceful Pregnancy

During pregnancy, the mother continues to eat an organic diet that is full of life and color—organic vegetables and fruit, antibiotic-free and hormone-free chicken and eggs, occasional free-range meat, and wild Alaska salmon. Because of the possibility of excessive levels of mercury in most fish, especially canned tuna, she pays special attention to the type of fish she eats. (Chapter 11 will give you an optimum diet for any stage of life.)

Our new mother is given special exercises for pregnancy by her midwife; she receives regular massages; and she dreams and meditates about the wondrous life that has been entrusted to her. She and her partner visualize a healthy, happy child that can have a full, meaningful, and productive life. The home environment is safe and secure and is free of cigarette smoke and toxic cleaning products. The baby's room was painted with water-based paints while the mother was away from the house for several days, to make sure she did not breathe in any harmful fumes.

Doulas and Delivery

The delivery takes place in a birthing center. It is attended by a doula (birth coach) and two midwives, with obstetricians nearby in case of any emergency. Because the mother practiced proper exercises during pregnancy and took Lamaze classes with instruction on breathing and relaxation, the birth is effortless. It's a girl! Her

Apgar score is 9, and she's just gorgeous. Her name? It's Zorra. Tears of joy! The abstinence from chemicals from preconception through delivery has achieved the intended goal of reducing the amount of xenoestrogen (chemicals that mimic estrogens) that the growing fetus was exposed to.

Puberty and Pubic Hairs

Zorra is a healthy child who rarely gets sick, eats well, takes supplements that her mother gives her, and is active in sports, theater, and dance. Her weight is normal for her height, and her skin is clear and her eyes sparkle with life.

Let's fast forward to puberty: Our young princess is now eleven years old, and she is showing signs of breast development and counting her pubic hairs! She's been waiting several years for this to happen, as most of her friends began developing long before and are already having their periods. Zorra's period begins when she is twelve; because she's been hearing about it from her friends for years, it doesn't come as a surprise.

Painless Periods

What does surprise Zorra about her period is her avoidance of cramps, crankiness, or heavy bleeding. Each month for two years, she has seen one of her friends go to the school nurse with nausea, vomiting, and severe stomach cramps. Zorra thought this was what periods were all about. Her friend, at age twelve, has a steady boyfriend and just went on the BCP to control her symptoms. Another friend has periods only every few months and was put on the pill because they were so irregular. Both friends talk about boys all the time, while Zorra is more interested in other extracurricular activities. Another girl in her class hasn't had her period yet; she is an intense athlete and is rumored to be anorexic.

Passing on the Pill

By age eighteen, Zorra is definitely interested in boys—young men, actually. She's a freshman in college, and she has decided it is time for her to join her friends and go on the pill. Interestingly enough, within a week of taking it she develops nausea, breast tenderness, and a feeling of irritation. When she asks her friends about this, they say they don't really feel any different on the pill but do remember feeling those symptoms in the beginning. They tell her she'll get used to it. But she says she doesn't want to get used to something that is making her feel lousy. Zorra can't help but notice that most of the girls in the dorm are overweight and complain regularly about fatigue and aches and pains, and that they are often sick with colds, flus, and stomach upsets. Zorra, on the other hand, is in great shape; she plays sports, does well in her subjects, and is usually in perfect health.

Zorra decides to call her aunt, an integrative medicine doctor, about her symptoms on the pill. Together, they decide that Zorra is being affected by the estrogen in the pill. By this time, a month has gone by; her first "period" on the days off the pill was very weak and the blood was brown and stringy.

Zorra has always been fascinated by her hormones and the monthly cycle that followed the moon. She has read everything she could about them, perhaps because she had waited so long for hers to come. Her knowledge gives her a great deal of respect for this miraculous process, and she decides that she doesn't want to artificially interfere with it. She realizes that she doesn't like the feeling of having too much estrogen and that she especially didn't like the change in her period. She decides to stop taking the pill. Instead, she takes a fertility course to learn how to read her vaginal and cervical mucus to identify the days when she is fertile. She uses this method as a means of contraception, along with condoms to avoid sexually transmitted disease that seemed to be rampant on campus.

Planning Her Pregnancy

When Zorra meets the man she will eventually marry, she has just graduated from her fine arts program and started a job illustrating at a publishing house. They both want to have children—and the sooner the better! Zorra's friends are all putting off pregnancy while they focus on their careers, but Zorra knows that she is at her peak of health and she doesn't want to waste it on late-night parties. She knows that she is more fortunate than some, because her career allows her to work from home part-time and, along with her husband, take care of a family as well.

Zorra and her husband follow the same plan that her parents had before she was born. The first time they try to get pregnant they are successful. Zorra is shocked! Just as she was shocked about her effortless periods, she is amazed at how easy it was for her to get pregnant. Her new friends and acquaintances at the publishing house are always talking about infertility problems. Women who had been on the pill for ten or fifteen years now find that they can't get pregnant. Some have had to have surgery to remove adhesions in their fallopian tubes from previous infections. Many have needed to take massive doses of fertility drugs to stimulate their body to get pregnant. Zorra considers herself very lucky. But her mother and aunt remind her that she has always taken good care of herself; if everyone else did the same, their experiences could be like hers.

Missing Menopause

Time whizzes by, and Zorra is now a healthy fifty years of age. Her periods for the past two years have been getting lighter and then have stopped. She has had a few hot flashes that just helped warm her up in winter, but nothing remarkable. Compared to her friends of the same age—many of whom have had ten years of peri-menopausal symptoms, fibroids, heavy bleeding, hysterectomies, and HRT—she again considers herself very fortunate. To keep her vaginal mucosa healthy and moist (as sex with her husband is very important to her), she adds some phytoestrogen herbs to her supplement program and gets a prescription for a very low-dose estriol vaginal cream from her doctor.

•••

And so it goes. Yeah, right, in a perfect world it goes this way, you say—not in the world that I live in. It's true; living such a completely balanced and harmonious life does seem out of our grasp. But once we know the causes of our problems, we can then work out their solutions. Read on, sort out for yourself your own imbalances, and then apply the solutions that are right for you.

What's Happening to My Hormones?

We ask this question in adolescence when we have irregular periods . . . in our twenties when we're hit with PMS or endometriosis . . . during pregnancy when mood swings and food cravings are easily blamed on rocketing hormones . . . and again in menopause when any and all symptoms are blamed on "the change." But nobody seems to know what's really going on. Let's go through the typical pattern of life stages, the ones we are more familiar with, the ones that many women complain about—the her-moanal years! Unfortunately, for many women these difficult her-moanal years start at first menses and continue right to menopause.

Early Puberty: Breasts at Ten, Moms at Twelve

A naturopathic doctor in Nova Scotia told me of an instance of pubescent fertility that shocked her community a few years ago.

Three twelve-year-old girls became pregnant by the same twelve-year-old boy. As they were obviously sexually mature at the age when they should still be playing with dolls, these children are now mothers.

An article on early puberty that appeared in a medical journal in 2004 demonstrates how pervasive this problem is.[1] According to the shocked researchers, "Nearly half of all black girls and 15 percent of white girls are beginning to develop sexually at the age of eight." A normal occurrence during puberty is a period of rapid growth and weight gain. One question that should be asked about the tremendous increase in obesity in children is whether sexual development comes before or after the weight gain.

An even more frightening statistic from this article states that 3 percent of black girls and 1 percent of white girls show signs of sexual development as early as three years of age. Compare this to an average age of menses onset at age sixteen-and-one-half years in 1835; at fourteen years in 1900; and at almost thirteen years in 1980.[2] Other researchers have estimated that the North American age of menses has decreased by three to four months each decade after 1850; in 1988 the median age at menarche was twelve-and-one-half years among American girls.[3]

Obesity and Early Puberty

Dr. Rose Frisch has been studying body fat and menses for decades. She says that the reason for the earlier onset of menses is pretty straightforward—it's all about the fat.[4] In her opinion, the body fat level at the onset of menses has remained relatively constant since 1840. Not many people realize that adipose (fat) cells have the ability to convert precursor hormones into estrogen (more on this in Chapter 4). What this means for overweight girls, however, is that they will start menstruating early. When I was in medical school, we were taught that the magic number was 100 pounds. When a young girl reaches that weight, she triggers off sequences of hormonal stimuli that will lead to puberty.

We also know that strenuous training for sports or dance can delay puberty by lowering body fat. So, just as 100 pounds is the trigger to start hormonal cycling, once you begin your periods and your weight falls below 100 pounds, your periods can stop. This doesn't mean that at 99.9 pounds something automatically turns off, but a dramatic drop in weight really can trigger hormonal shutdown. The lack of body fat signals the brain to turn off ovulation. Also, the body needs a certain amount of fat in the form of cholesterol in order to make hormones in the first place.

Dr. Marcia Herman-Giddens, the lead author of the paper on puberty mentioned above, says her team has no explanation for their findings that black girls are entering puberty approximately one to one-and-a-half years earlier than white girls and beginning menstruation approximately eight-and-a-half months earlier. However, taking a cue from Dr. Frisch and her work on fat and puberty, we may note that black girls have a higher incidence of overweight and obesity than white girls. According to one study, 36 percent of black children from age six to eleven are overweight, and 20 percent are obese; for white children of that age, the figures are 26 percent overweight and 12 percent obese.[5] That means that 20 percent of black girls might be expected to hit puberty early, compared to 12 percent of white girls. As Dr. Frisch demonstrated in 1970, it's the weight that determines when menses begins, not the chronological age.

More Culprits

The increase in obesity in children is one reason for the early onset of menses. How can we change that picture? For one thing, instead of just giving children earlier sex education, we need to take better care of their diet. Getting soda and other drinks sweetened with high-fructose corn syrup out of the school is the first step. Cutting back on junk food and introducing more vegetables and fruit to children's diets is the second.

Other culprits that are being targeted as triggers of early puberty are cosmetics—especially hair products that actually contain estrogen or placenta. We discuss such xenoestrogens and endocrine-disrupting chemicals in Chapter 6. These chemicals include pesticides, herbicides, and insecticides; growth hormones in meat; bovine growth hormone in milk; estrogen-like compounds used by dentists on children; and even the plastic wrap used on sandwiches for school lunches. The way to decrease the intake of chemicals is to encourage the use of organic food and discourage the use of processed and packaged food; we'll also speak more about diet in Chapter 11.

Sex in the Media

In her book *The Ageless Woman*, Dr. Serafina Corsello reminds us of another stimulus to early puberty.[6] Trained as a psychiatrist and practicing as an integrative medicine doctor, Corsello feels that the constant media images of sex and sexuality can be a sexual turn-on to young children and prematurely stimulate their sexual hormones. Sex research shows that images of erotica stimulate sexual hormonal release.

✄ The Birth Control Pill: Interfering with Nature

In my own case, I certainly appreciated being able to use the BCP for ten years in my life. It became so routine I didn't even think about it, even though I was practicing nutritional medicine and avoided taking drugs in general. Then one day a shiatsu practitioner said something to me about the energy to my ovaries being blocked. When I mentioned I was on the pill, he suggested that I consider other forms of birth control. Luckily, at the time I was taking regular supplements, which had probably prevented the vitamin B_6 and zinc deficiencies that are common with the pill. I then realized that I had been on the BCP for about ten years, which, according to my professors in medical school, is the maximum amount of time that you want to be on a synthetic hormone.

I later realized that when I started the pill I was put on the very high-dose pill that was common in the late 1960s, one that was still used in the mid-1970s. I was never given a lower dose—I never even thought about asking for one! I didn't seem to suffer any immediate effects while taking the pill (such as nausea, headache, or blood clots). However, I did not want to push my luck and take HRT, which would add to my estrogen load. Some women weren't as fortunate as I was with the BCP. Several years later, I wrote a journal article on PMS with a pharmacist friend. She was only in her mid-thirties, has been on the BCP for about ten years and suffered a paralyzing stroke that was blamed on the pill. It is one of the side effects that are listed for birth control pills, but most women aren't aware of this potentially lethal result.

Avoiding Pregnancy at What Cost?

A woman's first brush with synthetic hormones usually comes with adolescence. Either because of a desire for sexual intimacy or due to painful or irregular periods, we find ourselves on the BCP. Although cramping and painful periods may be due to a deficiency of progesterone and an excess of estrogen, many doctors prescribe the pill (which is usually estrogen-dominant) to alleviate painful symptoms. That's why some women have intolerable estrogen-induced side effects on the pill—such as weight gain, mood swings, and breast tenderness—even though their painful periods have been effectively suppressed.

Two Types of BCP

The birth control pill is the foundation of a $2.8 billion industry that is based on fooling sixteen million women's bodies into thinking and acting like they are pregnant. BCPs, or oral contraceptives, come in two forms. The *combined BCP* is a combination of two synthetic hormones—estrogen and progestin. The *minipill* consists solely of progestin (synthetic progesterone).

Combined BCPs are used the most, perhaps because they have been around the longest. The combination pill prevents ovulation from occurring by suppressing the natural hormones in the body that would stimulate the ovary to release an egg. Without an egg, pregnancy cannot occur. The estrogen part of the BCP makes sure that no egg will be developed or released for that month. Progestin acts to thicken the cervical mucus, which makes it difficult for the sperm to travel up the cervix. Progestin also prevents the lining of the uterus from developing normally; for this reason, even if an egg were fertilized, implantation would be unlikely.

The minipill only contains progestin, but in larger amounts that suppress ovulation as well as preventing sperm from navigating the cervix and keeping the uterus lining from developing.

No More Periods!

The latest version of oral contraceptives is a three-month pill called Seasonale—"the daily birth control that lets you have just four periods a year." Women are advised to take it for eighty-four days and then pause for a seven-day break to shed the buildup of blood vessels in the uterine lining. However, during a 2003 teleconference I attended, the makers of Seasonale said that women may even just have a two-day break from taking it. They expected that within three to five years this way of taking the pill would really catch on and about 50 percent of women taking the BCP would be on a continuous regimen.

The "experts" even advised that women who did not want to be bothered by their period could use a "monophasic" pill and *never* stop taking it. Monophasic simply means that there is the same dosage of hormone in every pill. No attempt is made to mimic the normal hormonal cycle—low estrogen and very low progesterone at the beginning of the cycle, a dip of estrogen at midcycle, and then an elevation of both estrogen and progesterone followed by an abrupt drop of both that heralds the period. Then the whole cycle starts all over again. The makers of Seasonale reminded the doctors on the conference call that there's no medical reason to have a period when you're on the pill because you're not getting a *real* period anyway.

No, the BCP is by no means a natural period created by an egg being formed in the ovary. There are no eggs being formed, because the pill makes your body believe it is already pregnant and shuts down the normal cycling of hormones. However, continuous use of the pill has not been sufficiently studied. We have no idea what the long-term effects of daily hormones will do to fertility or to other aspects of our health.

BCP Side Effects

We do, however, know some of the possible shorter-term effects of the BCP. The side effects of the combined pill, according to the manufacturer, include:

- Irregular bleeding or spotting
- Nausea
- Breast tenderness
- Weight gain and/or water retention
- Spotty darkening of the skin
- Mood changes

- Migraines
- Blood clots—thrombophlebitis and arterial thrombo-embolism
- Pulmonary embolism
- Strokes—cerebral hemorrhage, cerebral thrombosis
- Hypertension
- Heart attack—myocardial infarction
- Gallbladder disease
- Hepatic adenomas, or benign liver tumors

Nutritional Side Effects of the BCP

What is not usually mentioned is that the metabolism of BCPs by the liver requires extra amounts of the B-complex vitamins, vitamin C, magnesium, and zinc. This means that during all the years we took BCPs, we were creating nutrient deficiencies. Weight gain, fluid retention, mood changes, depression, and even heart disease can all arise from such nutrient imbalances. For example, we now know from decades of research that high levels of an amino acid called homocysteine cause heart disease. And high homocysteine occurs when there is a deficiency of B vitamins and magnesium.

Yeast Infections

The yeast Candida albicans makes its natural home in the gastro-intestinal tract. However, under the influence of a variety of factors—the BCP, antibiotics, cortisone, a highly refined bread and sugar diet, and stress—the yeast are encouraged to overgrow, and their toxins and their byproducts can adversely affect the whole body and not just local vaginal areas.

The symptoms range from headaches, head congestion, depression, and anxiety to throat and chronic cold symptoms, swollen glands, coated tongue, gastric upset, gas and bloating, constipation or diarrhea, vaginitis, arthritis, cystitis, muscle and joint aches, and numbness and tingling of the extremities. The symptoms are so widespread that it is sometimes difficult for an individual or her doctor to even comprehend that it could be a symptom complex.

Treating Yeast

The medical answer to vaginal yeast infections is local antifungal creams. Sometimes yeast infections are misdiagnosed, and antibiotics are given that only make the problem worse. Before going to antifungal medications, I have often recommended that patients use boric acid douches or boric acid suppositories as a local treatment for vaginal yeast infections. One teaspoon of boric acid dissolved in a pint of water in a douche bag is the recommended dosage. It's best to use water that is sterilized by boiling for twenty minutes, cooling it down and then adding the boric acid.

I also advise that my patients follow a diet that is very strict for the first few weeks in avoiding sugar, bread with yeast, fruit, fermented foods, and often most grains. Most people with the infection known as candidiasis report that they begin to feel much better by the second or third week. The first week can present some feeling of aggravation of symptoms if the yeast that are dying off flood the system and cause more symptoms than before. After several weeks on a strict diet, a reintroduction of foods would indicate whether you should in fact be consuming that food, which can represent either a food allergy or perhaps a yeast-promoting food.

The next step in treating a yeast infection is to add acidophilus bacteria to your diet. Acidophilus is a good bacteria that helps build up the normal flora in the bowel as the yeast are being killed off. Eating antifungal foods such as garlic and taking a tea called LaPacho or Teehebo can help kill yeast, as can caprylic acid made from coconut oil. Prescription medications such as Nystatin or Nizoral are used if symptoms remain.

✿ Stepping Up to the Gene Pool and Doing the Belly Flop

I am convinced that taking the BCP for ten and fifteen years is also contributing to the epidemic of infertility in young women. With a medical diagnosis of infertility invariably comes "fertility drugs." When I was in practice I had very few patients come to me with problems of infertility. When they did, diet, supplements, treating both partners, and emotional support usually did the trick. However, in the past dozen years that I've been researching, consulting, and writing, the rates of infertility have soared. I've consulted on many such cases; invariably, the keys to fertility were found in treating underlying infections and advising proper diet, supplements, and exercise. I'm the first to admit, though, that this doesn't work for everyone, and that's where allopathic medicine and fertility drugs come into the picture.

We Are the Experiment

Keep in mind that we really don't know what the sum total of BCP, fertility drugs, and HRT will do to the female body. This is not the kind of study that will be done by a drug company; it is, however, a study that many women are involved in simply through taking hormones throughout their lives. When gynecologists are asked if the BCP is a factor in infertility, they hedge and say probably not. Some will say that there are no studies to show that the BCP is associated with infertility. This may be true, but have such studies ever been attempted?

Let's look at what we do know. If a young girl has irregular periods, she is often offered the BCP to "regulate" them before she has even established a normal cycle. Ten years later, when that young woman and her partner want to become pregnant, she is simply told to go off the pill but wait three to six months for her own cycles to become regulated. If she doesn't become pregnant—without ever being given suggestions for an improved lifestyle, a better diet, or supplementary nutrients—the couple is sent to a "fertility" expert who begins a long series of tests and treatments that usually culminate in fertility drugs.

✳ Fertility Drugs

These very strong hormones may have long-term effects that are not yet recognized. For example, I'm hearing from women who have been treated with fertility drugs and are now experiencing extremely early menopause. The fertility drugs on the market are mostly focused on improving one thing—ovulation. As you will learn in Chapter 4, anovulatory cycles (a cycle that skips ovulation and goes straight to the period) are most common in puberty and perimenopause. The modern practice of delaying childbirth by suppressing ovulation—sometimes for ten or fifteen years with the BCP—may result in lack of proper synchronization of the hypothalamus and pituitary hormones that direct ovulation. Many young people are going on the pill during the first year of their cycles before they have become fully established. Other conditions that cause anovulatory cycles seem to be related to estrogen dominance, a condition we'll discuss in Chapter 4.

Drugs, given to women, are usually the first treatment option for couples who are determined to overcome their fertility problems. The two main drugs used are:

- *Clomiphene (Clomid),* which stimulates the hypothalamus and pituitary to trigger the release of eggs from the ovaries.
- *Gonadotropins,* which directly stimulate the ovaries to produce eggs.

Nature normally only allows one egg to grow and be released each month, but these drugs promote several eggs at one time. This increases the changes of pregnancy but also the chances of multiple births—10 percent on Clomid and 10 to 40 percent on gonadotropins. I have never seen a study that determines the long-term side effects of fertility drugs; my suspicion is that they help to deplete the thyroid and adrenal glands by putting extra pressure on the hypothalamus, pituitary, and ovaries.

The Thyroid and Adrenal Factor

Overactive, underactive, and inflamed are the three conditions that the thyroid can find itself in, and medical treatments are available for each situation. The adrenal glands, located above each kidney, are not diagnosed as over- or underactive until they are completely exhausted. Chapter 3 will discuss the important role of these two hormone glands in balancing our sex hormones.

Women Behaving Badly—PMS

Premenstrual syndrome (PMS) is defined as a combination of physical and emotional symptoms that occurs a week or ten days premenstrually, but that is absent the rest of the cycle. In some cases, the symptoms are severe enough to significantly interfere with work, family, or home activities. When I was in practice, I followed the work of Dr. Katrina Dalton, a British doctor who pioneered the use of progesterone for the treatment of severe PMS. At that time, in the early 1980s, the only way to administer progesterone was by injection or by rectal suppository. Oral progesterone was rapidly broken down in the liver and rendered useless. I chose the suppository route and found a compounding pharmacist to make up the medications. In 1986, I wrote a paper on PMS for the *Canadian Family Physician* that described the successful method of treating it with diet, supplements, and the occasional use of progesterone.[7]

Premenstrual dysphoric disorder (PMDD) is a condition that encompasses severe depression, irritability, and tension before menstruation. It appears to be a continuum of PMS with symptoms that are more severe. PMDD is actually a newly proposed mental disorder that has been officially accepted by the American Psychiatric Association (APA), and it is listed in the appendix of the APA's "bible," the Diagnostic and Statistical Manual of Mental Disorders, 4th edition (DSM-IV).

In a 2001 WebMD article entitled "Women Behaving Badly?"[8] the author talks about how Eli Lilly has marketed a product called Sarafem, intended for the treatment of PMDD. The package insert quotes heavily from the American Psychiatric Association's DSM-IV where PMDD is listed under "Mood Disorders Not Otherwise Specified."

This is not to disparage women with PMS, as I was one of the first doctors to recognize it and treat it. But the way to do so is not with a vamped-up Prozac in new packaging, which is what Sarafem is. According to the Sarafem Web site, the drug is meant to "help you be more like the woman you are, every day of the month, even during your most difficult days"; this is in spite of the fact that the Food and Drug Administration (FDA) advised (as quoted in the above 2001 WebMD article) that "the drug should be used only to treat women whose symptoms are severe enough to interfere with functioning at work or school, or with social activities and relationships."

WebMD interviewed Dr. Madeline Dehrendt, vice chairwoman of the Council on Women's Health of the World Chiropractic Alliance. She said, "From the time you're a preteen, from your very first inklings of hormonal rhythms all the way to the end of life, you're given the message that your body doesn't work or that it's not OK." Dr. Dehrendt recently spoke on this issue at the United Nations

Women's Conference, where, she says, she found that people all over the world appear to share her concerns.

Allyne Rosenthal, D.C., a Chicago-based chiropractor and functional medicine practitioner, is doubly concerned about the American Psychiatric Association's classification of PMS and the use of a drug such as Serafem on the teenage female population. She says, "The hallmark of adolescence is hormonal imbalance. Therefore, the numbers of young girls who will [be] deemed to be candidates for this medication are astronomical if they go ahead with this, and that is one of the major problems."

A woman after my own heart, Dr. Rosenthal says, "The vision of millions of women being put on this drug for a condition that can be so effectively treated in other ways is just stunning. PMS is something that bothers a lot of women. There's no question about that, but it responds incredibly well—and quickly—to a combination of things, like vitamin B_6, magnesium, zinc, and the correct balance of proteins and carbohydrates in the diet."

Nada Stotland, M.D., M.P.H., is a professor of psychiatry and obstetrics and gynecology at Rush Medical College in Chicago, and a member of a task force that determined the DSM-IV diagnostic criteria. Dr. Stotland told WebMD that she argued against including PMDD in the main text of the manual. She also makes the observation that there is a spike in driving accidents with teenage boys and that the adolescent surge of testosterone is probably to blame. But no one is asking teenage boys to take drugs to keep them and everyone else safe. "So which is worse: being crabby or being run over?" she quips. She is also a realist when she says, "In terms of PMDD, I think the evidence speaks for itself. Prozac's patent was running out, and suddenly a new disorder appeared—PMDD—that changed the classification to mental disorders. So with that a new class was formed, a new market was formed, and a new patent was formed."

✦ Perimenopause and Menopause

When I began hearing about perimenopause, I wondered if part of the symptoms we see in women leading up to menopause could be attributed to progesterone deficiency. You'll read in Chapter 8 about Dr. Jerilynn Prior's discovery that perimenopausal women actually have higher estrogen levels than normal. This means that progesterone may then be relatively lower than estrogen and be responsible for creating symptoms of hormone imbalance.

Menopause is another normal life event that has been medicated with HRT since the 1960s. In the 1980s we learned that estrogen in the form of Premarin (from pregnant mare's urine), when used for twenty years to treat symptoms of menopause, was causing uterine cancer. Immediately, drug companies promoted a combined synthetic estrogen and synthetic progesterone (progestin) HRT treatment for menopause, saying that the progestin component would protect the uterus. Finally, in 2003, a huge research trial was terminated halfway through the study when it was found that adding the progestin to synthetic estrogen did not protect the uterus and actually caused a higher incidence of breast cancer. Neither did the combined HRT prevent heart attack, osteoporosis, Alzheimer's, or senility, as many medical experts had promised.

Surgical Menopause

Removal of the uterus for fibroids, excessive bleeding, or endometriosis is one of the most common surgical procedures in America. In fact, according to a report by Dr. Adrienne Fugh-Berman, one third of women have had a hysterectomy before reaching menopause.[9] Along with removal of the uterus, there often comes the unnecessary amputation of the ovaries—unnecessary because it's often not done for any disease of the ovaries but as a "preventive" measure against ovarian cancer. Such sudden elimination of a woman's major source of estrogen and progesterone sends her into immediate menopause with hot flashes, fatigue, and mood swings. The only treatment given to women in the throes of menopausal symptoms has been synthetic estrogen. We'll discuss natural hormone supplements in Chapter 12, and, the safer bioidentical HRT in Chapter 13.

✂ NaPro Technology: The Alternative to the BCP and Much More

When I was in private practice I introduced my female patients to methods that would help them understand the physical changes caused by their hormones. These methods were also the standard methods of natural contraception that were embraced by a generation of women who did not want to use the BCP, yet still wanted control over their own reproduction.

I now recommend the Creighton Model Fertility Care System (CrM). It uses the science-based method of NaPro Technology (NaPro), a women's health science that evolved from physiological interpretation of the biomarkers of the menstrual and fertility cycle. The underlying premise is to understand your fertility and gynecological health by learning how to evaluate easily accessed biological markers.

These biological markers are, mainly, cervical mucus score, the length and intensity of the menstrual flow, and the length of the pre– and post–Peak phase (the Peak Day itself being the chief indicator of ovulation). Such markers are exquisitely sensitive to the dance of hormones in the body. Learning CrM and using NaPro allows both the woman and her doctor to understand what's happening in the menstrual cycle and to reach the correct "diagnosis" and eventual cooperative treatments. If there is too much estrogen, it shows up in the cervical mucus. If there is too little progesterone, that too shows up as a change in the cervical mucus.

Premenstrual or postmenstrual brown bleeding, spotting, or short post–Peak phase are just a few of the signs that are observed. This is an invaluable technique for diagnosing infertility, anovulatory cycles, and the cause of perimenopausal symptoms. Once a woman is able to NaPro her cycle, she can work with a doctor familiar with the NaPro Technology. Together they are able to

- Identify chronic discharges.
- Evaluate hormones and apply appropriate hormonal treatment (with bioidentical hormones).
- Identify functional ovarian cysts and treat them nonsurgically by using the appropriate bioidentical hormone.
- Evaluate the effects of stress.
- Treat premenstrual syndrome.
- Evaluate, treat, and/or prevent reproductive abnormalities such as infertility, miscarriage, ectopic pregnancy, stillbirth, and prematurity.
- Identify and treat perimenopause.
- Evaluate and treat heavy uterine bleeding and help avoid hysterectomy by applying the appropriate hormonal treatment.

You can learn more about NaPro Technology at *www.naprotechnology.com.*

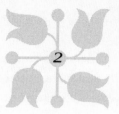

Broken Promises:
The History of HRT

IT'S ONLY IN THE PAST one hundred years, since the lifespan of women has almost doubled, that we have been able to focus on menopause and what it means to women. We'll discuss more about how menopause is viewed in different countries in Chapter 9. In this chapter I want to give the history of HRT and how menopause came to be called a disease. According to modern medicine, labeling menopause a disease meant a drug had to be found to "cure" it.

The Timeline of HRT

The Hormone Foundation, an independent, nonprofit organization established by the Endocrine Society in 1997, offers a credible timeline of hormonal advances in the past century. (You can find this timeline online at *www.hormone.org/publications/estrogen_timeline/*.) The writing of the timeline was made possible due to an "unrestricted grant" given by Wyeth Pharmaceuticals, the makers of Premarin. My timeline is a heavily edited version of theirs.

Living Longer with Hormones

As it states in the preamble to the Hormone Foundation timeline: "In the past century, medical advances have helped extend women's lives by more than 35 years. The average woman can now expect to live more than 80 years. Estrogen may play a role in maintaining health and well-being throughout these years. The isolation of estrogen in 1929 was the first of many steps in the development of today's oral contraceptives and hormone therapies."

Menopause Is Born

In 1821, a century before the isolation of estrogen, a French physician named de Gardanne invented the term menopause to describe the phenomenon of this transition phase in a woman's life and the problems thereof. (His book was titled *De la ménopause, ou de l'âge critique des femmes*, which might be translated as *On Menopause, or The Critical Age for Women*.) Over the next 100 years, many researchers around the world searched for the "cure." In the late 1800s, doctors experimented with testicular extracts for men and ovarian extracts for women. It wasn't until the early 1900s that doctors realized that the ovaries produce two hormones, later called estrogen and progesterone.

Contraception Research

Inhibiting fertility was a focus of much research, and the first positive results were reported in 1919. Subcutaneous implants of ovaries from pregnant rabbits were injected into deer, rendering them infertile. It took eight years more of research to achieve temporary sterility in mice by using oral ovarian extracts.

Progesterone contraception reached a successful conclusion in 1937 when researchers at the University of Pennsylvania were able to prevent ovulation in a rabbit. Over the next several decades several synthetic estrogens and progestins were developed.

In 1956 Planned Parenthood funded the first controlled trial with a contraceptive pill containing norethynodrel. But in 1957 Enovid, the norethynodrel-containing oral contraceptive, was approved and marketed only for the treatment of menstrual disturbances, and not as an oral contraceptive. In 1960 the FDA approved the use of Enovid as the first oral contraceptive pill specifically to prevent pregnancy. In 1964 the second oral contraceptive, ethinyl estradiol, was approved by the FDA, and by 1965 there were already more than 2.3 million oral contraceptive users.

Curing Menopause

In 1929, the first American doctors to attempt to treat menopause symptoms were Drs. E. L. Severinghaus and J. Evans. Their treatment of choice was a derivative from the amniotic fluid of cattle. In 1930, a German doctor, Bernhard Zondek found that urine from pregnant mares contained water-soluble estrogens. Other researchers realized that decomposed and hydrolyzed pregnant mare's urine contained estradiol.

By 1933, a product made from the urine of pregnant women, Emmenin (which contained water-soluble estrogens, but mostly estriol glucuronide), became the first estrogen replacement product marketed in the United States. But work began immediately on producing a less expensive version from pregnant mare's urine.

In 1939, diethylstilbestrol (DES) was marketed as a more potent form of estrogen than Emmenin. By 1948, it was advertised as having therapeutic value for the prevention of pregnancy complications, such as toxemia, low birth weight, and early pregnancy loss. Approximately two million women were exposed to DES during pregnancy in those years. The text in major medical journals in the 1950s describing DES read, "Recommended for routine prophylaxis in ALL pregnancies

. . . Bigger and stronger babies . . . No gastric or other side effects." It wasn't until 1953 that a controlled trial using DES showed it had no clinical benefit in preventing complications during pregnancy.

By 1942 the higher-dose Premarin—1.25 milligrams—was introduced to the U.S. public. Six years later, in 1948, the lower doses of Premarin—0.625 milligram and 0.3 milligram—were made available. In the 1950s, Ayerst Laboratories funded a massive campaign to educate doctors on menopause, menopausal symptoms, and the consequences of estrogen loss—and on the use of its product Premarin to treat menopausal symptoms.

In the 1960s the use of estrogen replacement therapy (ERT) escalated to include about 12 percent of all postmenopausal women. Premarin use grew 170 percent from 1963 to 1966, and it became the #1 dispensed drug in America. The spurt in ERT use was given a boost in particular when Dr. Robert A. Wilson published his article "No More Menopause" in *Newsweek* magazine in January 1964.

⚘ Feminine Forever: The Marketing of Menopause

Spurred on by his popular article on menopause in *Newsweek* in 1964, Dr. Robert Wilson promised millions of women in his 1966 book that they could be *Feminine Forever*. In this book, he promoted estrogen to American women, and he widely educated women and doctors to believe that "Menopause is an estrogen-deficiency disease." By naming menopause a deficiency disease, the next step was to advise replacement therapy in the form of Premarin. The very basis of estrogen treatment belied the fact that producing lower levels of hormones with age is a normal part of life.

According to the *New York Times* in July 2002, Ronald Wilson reported that his father's research foundation, book, and speaking tours were funded by Wyeth-Ayerst, the makers of Premarin. I have a vintage copy of *Feminine Forever*, and I see no acknowledgment or disclosure that his promotion of estrogen was sponsored by Wyeth-Ayerst.

In his book, Dr. Wilson expresses his "sympathy" to women, who should not be "condemned to witness the death of their own womanhood" but who should be allowed to "remain fully feminine—physically and emotionally—for as long as they live." He lauded the major medical breakthrough that allowed women "the opportunity to remain a complete woman." He referred to himself as a "gallant knight" on a mission to help women through their "loss of womanhood." He even goes so far as to compare himself to Dr. Ignaz Semmelweiss, who, after examining women with severe postsurgical infections, urged fellow doctors to wash their hands before performing surgery. Semmelweiss's advice was ridiculed and he was fired and castigated. Wilson announced his frustration that the world was ignoring his "medical procedure of tremendous value to every woman." So what did he do? He went directly to the people—with the backing of the makers of Premarin, and without the necessary science to proceed—and he spearheaded an extensive experiment on women.

Much of the book is patriarchal and patronizing and very, very dated considering what woman have accomplished in the last forty years. Wilson even advises women to take Premarin to prevent their husbands from having extramarital affairs. His opinion: "In truth, an extramarital affair may not, in the literal sense of the term, involve any infidelity at all. For a man may loyally maintain a deep love for his wife and yet feel the need for a kind of thrill that a wife with her aura of comfortable domesticity cannot give." By some miracle, Premarin was supposed to change a housewife into a vamp who keeps her man. Please!

But the PR worked, and within ten years of the publication of *Feminine Forever*, Wyeth-Ayerst's Premarin was the fifth-leading prescription drug in America. Obviously, such commercial promotion under the guise of "friendly" advice from a trusted doctor is hardly "scientific"; it denies patients the right to proper scientific evidence of the harmful effects of estrogen, while only promoting the so-called benefits. Today, "friendly" promotion for HRT still appears in the form of commercial endorsements from popular singers and actresses, people whom the public admire and whose example they follow.

✎ Give Men Estrogen for Heart Disease

"If estrogen deficiency's a disease, all men have it!" says Dr. Susan Love, breast surgeon and author, who loves to take pot shots at the menopause industry. In fact, some researchers used men in the very first clinical trial to prove that estrogen prevented heart attacks. Researchers had long felt that women had less heart disease before menopause because of estrogen. Back in 1973, they were so sure that estrogen was associated with heart health that they enrolled a group of men and put them on estrogen. They were shocked to find that early in the trial those men on estrogen were experiencing more heart attacks than those on placebo. The trial had to be stopped. Instead of wondering if the same would occur in women, they just shrugged their shoulders and said that maybe the dose of estrogen was too high. As you'll read later, not until the 2003 analysis of the Women's Health Initiative study was there an admission that hormone replacement can, indeed, increase the risk of cardiovascular disease.

✎ Estrogen Side Effects Accumulate

By 1968 there were numerous reports of an increased risk of cardiovascular disease and strokes with the use of high-dose oral contraceptives. Within a few years, oral contraceptives containing less than 50 mcg ethinyl estradiol, when compared to those containing more than 50 mcg, showed a lower risk; many women switched to the lower dose pills. Studies of women on estrogen also revealed an increased incidence of endometrial cancer. By 1972 there was a moratorium on the use of estrogen, alone, for menopause. The shocking news that DES was causing an increase in cancer added fuel to the anti-estrogen lobby.

The DES Story

DES was pulled from the market in 1971 when babies born to DES users were found to have increased incidence of cancer of the reproductive organs. It has taken over thirty years, a whole generation, to come to this conclusion. In 1977 a DES registry was formed to collect information regarding the use of DES and to alert women who had used DES in their pregnancy to inform their children. DES children were developing genital tract lesions and gynecologic cancers in their adulthood.

Breast Cancer Surfaces

It wasn't until the late 1980s that reports of breast cancer with the continued use of ERT surfaced. We now know that breast cancer takes fifteen to twenty years to develop from its original inception. In the early 1990s tamoxifen, an estrogen receptor modulator, was touted first for treating and later for preventing breast cancer. It is being recommended to healthy women even though we have no idea of the long-term effects. What we do know, however, is that it was labeled a carcinogen in 1996. It has the unusual distinction of being able to cause and cure the same condition.

The Search for Benefits of ERT

With all the negative side effects of estrogen being reported, the pharmaceutical industry pushed to find some benefits. Several studies were reported in 1980. One study showed a 60 percent reduced risk of hip and wrist fractures in women taking ERT, another study showed inhibition of postmenopausal bone loss. Several studies implied that the risk of endometrial cancer could be reduced by adding a second hormone to the ERT regimen—synthetic progesterones called progestin. Epidemiologic reports of lessened cardiovascular risk with ERT also appeared at this time. By the late 1980s, estrogen became available as a transdermal patch. All in all, by the mid-1990s researchers had claimed that postmenopausal estrogen may be useful in the prevention of the following diseases: Alzheimer's disease, age-related eye disease, colon cancer, tooth loss, diabetes, and Parkinson's disease.

Estrogen on Trial

Several large-scale hormone trials were finally initiated to prove or disprove the safety of hormone replacement and its possible benefits:

- *The Heart Estrogen/Progestin Replacement Study (HERS).* Between February 1993 and September 1994, twenty HERS centers recruited and randomized 2,763 women to study estrogen in relation to heart disease.
- *The Women's Health Initiative (WHI) clinical trial and observational study,* sponsored by the National Institutes of Health, followed over 161,000 postmenopausal women for over ten years. The objective of the clinical trial was to evaluate the effects of postmenopausal estrogen use, dietary patterns, and calcium and vitamin D supplements on overall mortality, cardiovascular disease, breast cancer, colon cancer, osteoporosis, and other disease processes.
- *The Women's Health, Osteoporosis, Progestin, Estrogen Study (Women's HOPE Study)* evaluated the effects of low-dose HRT on menopausal symptoms and osteoporosis.

- *The British Million Women Study* looked into estrogen and pro-gestin effects in the largest group ever studied.
- New clinical trials on a selective estrogen receptor modula-tor (SERM)—the drug raloxifene—were begun. This drug is considered a second-generation SERM (after tamoxifen). Tri-als on osteoporosis prevention, heart disease prevention, and breast cancer prevention were initiated with this drug.

The Verdict on Estrogen

The news was increasingly unfavorable for ERT and HRT from the late 1990s onward. After estrogen was found to cause uterine cancer, the spate of trials in the 1980s showing some benefits of estrogen did not hold up under closer scrutiny and with much larger study populations.

1997: Data published in *The Lancet* (the British medical journal) from fifty-one epidemiological studies indicated an increased risk of breast cancer with postmenopausal estrogen use.[10]

1998: The Heart Estrogen/Progestin Replacement Study (HERS) found no heart benefit to women who took HRT and had cardiovascular disease. And women given HRT showed an increased risk of a second cardiovascular event during the first year on HRT compared to women given a placebo.

2002: The HERS study was extended and still showed no cardio-vascular benefit of HRT in postmenopausal women with previous history of cardiovascular disease.

2002: The estrogen/progestin portion of the WHI study originally scheduled to end in 2005 was halted because of an increased incidence of invasive breast cancer and an excess of risk vs. benefit. The study also showed a decreased risk of colorectal

cancer and fractures but an increased risk of venous thromboembolism.

2003: Further analysis of the WHI study indicated that there was
an increase in the risk of cardiovascular events and breast
cancer in women taking estrogen plus progestin.

The British Million Women study also found that women who
are taking estrogen/progestin increased the density of their breast
tissue. This may lead to incorrect mammogram readings and possibly make mammograms less reliable in detecting small cancers.

✳ Reaction to the Women's Health Initiative Announcement

As mentioned above, a full three years before the study was supposed to be completed the estrogen/progestin arm of the Women's
Health Initiative study had to be halted. Ethical review boards
constantly review statistics from studies, and in the WHI study it
became obvious that there was an increased incidence of invasive
breast cancer in the HRT group. There was also an increased risk of
thromboembolism—the formation of blood clots that can travel to
other parts of the body such as the brain and heart, causing stroke
or heart attack.

Often bad news in studies doesn't reach the public, but there
were no holds barred in reporting this distressing information. Over
six million American women were taking estrogen-progestin pills
in 2002. They, along with the doctors who were prescribing these
drugs, were shocked to hear that HRT was proving to be more harmful than beneficial. However, anyone keeping up on the literature
had seen the writing on the wall. The negative findings in the 1997
Lancet review and the 1998 report on HERS were only the tip of the
iceberg. Even with those studies, the message from HRT proponents

was always that we needed more studies and more proof. In July 2002 irrefutable proof was there for everyone to see.

Later analysis of the WHI results, published in May 2004, revealed that the risk of dementia doubled in women sixty-five and older who were taking HRT. Prompted by press releases and news reports that hormones might prevent Alzheimer's, many doctors began prescribing for this "off-label" condition. (Off-label means that a drug is prescribed for non-FDA–approved indications.)

WHI and Premarin Alone

Women who have had hysterectomies take Premarin without progestins and account for about eight million Premarin users. The Premarin-alone arm of the WHI study was allowed to continue until 2004. However, it too was prematurely halted in February 2004, because there was an increased risk of stroke, a significantly increased risk of deep vein thrombosis, and no observable benefit to coronary heart disease.

The only benefit was a reduced risk of hip and other fractures. However, when analyzing the actual bone fracture statistics, the report said that the increased benefit for the bones is based on a total of six fewer hip fractures. In the 10,739 women studied, there were eleven cases of hip fracture for women on Premarin and seventeen cases in women taking placebo. It is hard to see how these figures—involving only six people—can be called statistically significant results that allow the study authors to say that Premarin has a beneficial effect in preventing hip fractures.

Dr. Barbara Alving, acting director of the National Heart, Lung, and Blood Institute, said, "These findings confirm that Premarin-alone therapy should not be used to prevent chronic disease." She also said, "We believe the findings support current FDA recommendations that hormone therapy only be used to treat menopausal symptoms and that it be used at the smallest effective dose for the shortest possible time." Researchers remind women that the study's results are only evidence of what happens to women when they take continuous Premarin for 6.8 years.

✕ Why WHI Happened

Decades of advocating for women's health by grass-roots, feminist groups brought about the 1991 government-funded WHI study, according to Abby Lippman, professor of epidemiology at McGill University and co-chair of the Canadian Women's Health Network (CWHN).[11] In Dr. Lippman's opinion, "Women were concerned by the increasing medicalization of women's lives and by physicians' tendency to push 'pills for prevention' of everything from hot flashes to memory lapses." Lippman is a women's advocate who derives her remarks from communication with a variety of women's groups. She stated that women across North America "believed that federally-funded research was the only way to get results not tainted by pharmaceutical company interests, and they argued that this unbiased information was what women needed if they were to make informed decisions about their health."

Dr. Lippman also remarked, "Without the intervention of the U.S. National Women's Health Network and others, millions more would be getting prescriptions for HRT merely due to what the Network has called the 'triumph of marketing over science.'" Drug companies have been spending billions in advertising to doctors in Canada and the United States, and to the American public, lauding the wondrous effects of HRT. Beyond spreading the message that HRT is not going to prevent chronic disease, Dr. Lippman says, "Pills for healthy people can be dangerous! And the burgeoning advertisements and other marketing activities of pharmaceutical companies are serious, potentially lethal, threats to our well-being."

This is not just Dr. Lippman's opinion; many women who are approaching the magic age of fifty have noted the habitual response of doctors. One glance at your age, one ear to hear a few of your nonspecific complaints, a quick peek at their watch, and out comes a prescription pad for HRT.

WHI and the Stock Market

Bad news spreads faster on Wall Street than it does in doctors' offices. While many doctors remained equivocal about the results of the WHI study, it only took a few hours for the stock market to react. Shares of Wyeth, the makers of the $2 billion dollar drug (in 2001 sales) used in the study, fell by 19 percent. The company's public relations team responded to the news by emphasizing that it was the combination pill of Premarin and progestin (Prempro) that was at fault and not their Premarin.

Wall Street and WHI Premarin-Alone Study

By March of 2004, the Premarin-alone arm of the WHI study showed no ability to prevent heart disease and even showed a higher risk of stroke. According to one newspaper account, Wyeth heaved a sigh of relief because at least Premarin did not show an increase in breast cancer or heart attack as did the combination pill.[12] By giving investors this "encouraging" news, Wyeth prevented another stock market plunge. By the end of the day Wyeth stock was only down 11 percent from two years earlier, before the first announcement about Prempro. In actual sales figures, for the drugs themselves, sales of Prempro fell from $888 million in 2001 to $292 million in 2003. In the same two-year period, Premarin sales fell from $1.2 billion to $984 million.

The findings of the Premarin arm of the WHI study could still change, however, since women in the study will be followed until 2007. It must be remembered that it takes fifteen to twenty years for cancer to develop; the WHI trial only began in 1991 and it really should run until 2011. We also know that women have been taking Premarin since the 1950s, paralleling the increased incidence of breast cancer.

Healthier Women Choose Premarin

In a 2002 interview, Dr. Marcia Stefanick of Stanford University, who led the team of researchers on the WHI study, said the results of the WHI study would not necessarily reflect the general population because of overwhelming evidence in past decades that "estrogen users were by and large a healthier group of women, and so we have what we call the healthy user bias effect [leading to] the incorrect belief that estrogen or estrogen and progestins would prevent heart disease."[13] Dr. Stefanick also noted that women who take hormones are also more likely to take better care of themselves through diet, exercise, and keeping their weight down. She commented that these are the approaches that "we now would like to encourage women to recognize as a better approach to preventing heart disease." So, in fact, it may not be the hormones that prevent heart disease as much as the diet and exercise habits of the women who take them.

No More Magic Bullets

Previously approved only for menopausal symptoms and osteoporosis prevention by the FDA, HRT has been promoted by drug companies as the magic bullet for many other conditions. Using the results of small industry-funded studies showing possible protective advantage in aging, cancer, and heart attacks, drug company reps were pushing HRT for off-label conditions. Essentially, we are back in the mid-1970s when researchers realized that estrogen alone was causing endometrial cancer, and we mustn't forget those decades-old results. Since that time, estrogen alone has only been recommended to women who have had a hysterectomy, as it is not an option for women who still have their uterus.

Dr. Victoria Kusiak, Wyeth's North American medical director, has stated, "We certainly think that the significant finding from the study was that there was no increased risk of breast cancer." As a physician, I do not gain confidence enough from this to recommend Premarin—though it does give me more confidence to suggest alternatives! We'll get to those alternatives, which include natural hormone replacement, in Chapters 11 to 13.

✂ Advice from the FDA

About a year and a half after the announcement that Prempro was doing more harm than good, and before we learned that Premarin was not as beneficial as some thought, the FDA launched a nationwide campaign "to provide better health information to women about the use of hormones to treat symptoms of menopause." The campaign was directed at the more than ten million women using ERT and HRT and the two million women per year who enter menopause. Six months after the Prempro study was halted, the FDA advised women and health care professionals that "menopausal hormone therapy is associated with an increased risk of heart disease, heart attacks, strokes, and breast cancer." The warning emphasized that these products are not approved for heart disease prevention. (Yes, this repeats what has been said above—the point is that the concern about the use of HRT expressed earlier is also the FDA's concern.)

The FDA's press release goes on to say that, "because there are few "proven" alternatives for the relief of hot flashes and vaginal atrophy, menopausal hormone therapies have an important role in women's health." But, hastens to add, "It is very important that women realize that this beneficial therapy also carries significant risks. Our recommendation is that if you choose to use hormone therapy for hot flashes or vaginal dryness, or if you prefer it to other treatments to prevent thin bones, take the lowest dose for the least duration required to provide relief." Labeling of hormones will also change and will "clarify that these drugs should be used only when the benefits clearly outweigh risks."

Questions to Ask Your Doctor, Nurse, or Pharmacist

The FDA provides a list of nine questions to ask your health care practitioner. Number two is: "Are there other things I can use or do?" But the FDA has already stated that "because there are few 'proven' alternatives for the relief of hot flashes and vaginal atrophy, menopausal hormone therapies have an important role in women's health."

Question nine asks, "Do you have any advice to help me: Exercise, Stop smoking, Eat right, Sleep better, Reduce stress?" There is no mention in any of the FDA's educational literature (which is paid for by taxpayers, by the way) is there any mention of the vitamin, mineral, herbal, homeopathic, or other non-drug therapies—many of which, in fact, have proven useful in menopause both in scientific studies and in ample anecdotal clinical cases.

Bailing on HRT

After the announcement about the dangers of HRT in July 2002, millions of women stopped their medications. From about six million users of combined therapy in 2002, by July 2003 there were only about 3.3 million. The number of women taking estrogen alone is estimated at about 6.7 million. In Chapters 11 and 12, we'll talk about the many foods and supplements that can help women with menopausal symptoms. In Chapter 13 we'll also discuss how natural HRT with bioidentical hormones may be the short-term therapy that has fewer side effects than synthetic HRT.

Measuring Breast Cancer Risk

Women in general, and especially women on HRT, are advised to have an annual mammogram. Mammograms are presently the diagnostic gold standard for breast cancer, but I predict that over the next decade medical thermography will take on that role. How does thermography work? When cancer cells begin dividing rapidly, the temperature of those cells increases ever so slightly. Thermography measures these temperature changes to 1/10,000th of a degree. It therefore has the potential to detect abnormal cells in breast tissue and tumors the size of a grain of rice, five to seven years before a lump can be felt when ½ inch in size, or even seen by mammography at 1/8 inch. With a thermogram, you avoid the 42 pounds per square inch pressure on sensitive breasts that has been known to damage breast tissue and spread cancer cells due to the pressure. You also avoid the risk of radiation from mammograms.

The only type of thermography that I recommend is Digital Infrared Imaging (DII). It requires two pictures, one before and one after a cold challenge where you put your hands in freezing water for one minute. A computer reads the difference in the two images and determines if there is an area of increased blood circulation and heat, which is a sign of abnormal growth. (See the Resources section for contact information.)

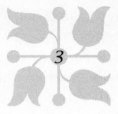

3

The Hormonal Sextet:
Hypothalamus, Pituitary, Thyroid, Parathyroids, Adrenals, Ovaries

TO CREATE THEIR SEX HORMONES, women need a sextet of endocrine glands working in concert, with the right amount of hormone reaching the right destination at the right time. Because hormones are secreted into the general blood circulation and reach all parts and all cells of the body, a cell must have a way to attract the specific hormone that it needs. When that happens, the right hormone reaches the right cell, and it gives the right message to parts of the cell called *receptor sites*. For example, when estradiol finds its corresponding receptor sites, it is able to do its job of increasing cell division. When it reaches receptor sites on the uterus, estradiol causes the endometrial lining to thicken; when it reaches breast receptor sites, it stimulates breast cells to grow. Basically, in order for any hormone to work it must be able to attach to a receptor in the targeted tissue. If one or more aspects of this orchestration are out of kilter, the message is lost—or, even worse, the message is distorted, resulting in an aberrant response.

According to Dr. Candace Pert, the author of *Molecules of Emotion*, a receptor is a molecule, made of protein, that is anchored in a cell's outer membrane in a site accessible to the environment external to the cell. The function of the receptor is to bind with *ligands* such as hormones, antigens, drugs, peptides, or neurotransmitters called "informational substances." Dr. Pert has found that the receptor is the key player in the body's communication network, because it is only when the receptor is occupied by the ligand that the message encoded in the informational substances can be received by the cell. (The word "ligand" is from the Latin word *ligare*, meaning "that which binds." It refers to a variety of small molecules that bind specifically to a cell receptor site and convey information to the cell.)

The way receptor sites act as guardians for any information getting into the body will be of particular importance when we later talk about xenoestrogens. These substances, as well as some other chemicals, can jam up receptor sites and pass along chaotic messages to the cell or make the cell receptors unavailable to receive the messages they need for survival.

Hormone Disharmony

When I was in medical school, the various hormones were taught separately, and I learned to divide them up into individual, discrete boxes. The major organs that produce hormones are the thyroid, ovaries, and adrenals. The thyroid seemed to be the organ that took up most of our classroom and study time. In cases where it became hyperactive, we learned to use drugs or surgery to destroy part of the gland. When it became hypoactive, we were taught to use thyroid replacement therapy. The thinking was similar for the female hormones, except that we were told that they did not become hyperactive, but would become hypoactive in menopause. The suggested treatment was estrogen replacement therapy.

I was also taught in medical school that the adrenal glands either function perfectly normally or else they become completely exhausted and cease to function, as in Addison's disease. Nothing was mentioned about any in-between stage. Having no adrenal gland function is a death sentence, but adrenal gland hormone replacement therapy can be given to someone with Addison's disease and they can lead a fairly normal life. Addison's disease is actually extremely rare, and I never ran across the condition in my practice. However, the sad truth is that the majority of women these days have adrenal insufficiency—especially women in menopause.

Some Definitions to Know

For those who haven't been to medical school, here are some definitions of terms related to hormones and glands:

Hormone: A chemical substance (also called a "messenger" molecule) produced in the body's endocrine glands that exerts a regulatory or stimulatory effect. One example: insulin, produced by the pancreas, promotes the uptake of glucose by body cells.

Endocrine: Glands that secrete hormones internally directly into the lymph or bloodstream.

Hypothalamus: A central area on the underside of the brain that secretes hormones that stimulate or suppress the release of hormones in the pituitary gland.

Pituitary: A small oval gland at the base of the brain producing the hormones that control the thyroid, adrenals, and ovaries; it also produces growth hormone, antidiuretic hormone, prolactin, and oxytocin.

Thyroid: An endocrine gland located in the neck that secretes thyroxin, triiodothyronine, and calcitonin, which control metabolic rate, body heat, and growth, including bone growth.

Ovaries: Female reproductive organs that produce eggs and secrete the sex hormones estrogen and progesterone.

Adrenals: Endocrine glands that are located above each kidney. The inner part (medulla) secretes catacholamine adrenaline (epinephrine) and noradrenaline (norepinephrine) that react to stress. The outer part (cortex) secretes hydrocortisone, androgen (male) hormones, and aldosterone, which affect blood pressure and salt balance.

Parathyroid: A gland that secretes a parathyroid hormone, which affects calcium levels in the blood.

Hormone Harmony

Hypothalamus, pituitary, thyroid, parathyroids, adrenals, and ovaries—six interacting players in a high-stakes hormonal game. Whatever is done by one of the players reverberates through the whole group. We can't really understand how the female hormones—estrogen and progesterone—work unless we explore the other players. The standard medical approach of simply giving synthetic estrogen and synthetic progesterone replacement therapy doesn't acknowledge the role played by the other endocrine glands in the body.

The feedback systems among these organs travel faster than any chemicals could possibly move; they therefore must be connected by the nervous system or some even speedier system that we have yet to discover. Most tissues in the body are also equipped with hormonal receptor sites that have a unique configuration to allow a specific hormone to be accepted into a particular tissue for a particular purpose. For example, the hormone insulin, which is secreted by the pancreas, responds to high blood glucose levels and unlocks cell membranes, opening them up to allow glucose to come into the cells.

Who's in Charge?

The hypothalamus and pituitary are the master glands that put the game of life in motion, as they control growth, metabolism, and sexual development. The thyroid, parathyroids, adrenals, and ovaries take orders from the master glands, but they also have a say in how much or how little hormones they produce. So, in fact, the endocrine system is an orchestration that requires all the players to be fully engaged. Besides the six already mentioned, the other endocrine glands—the pineal, pancreas, thymus, and placenta—also have important functions in the body that relate to sleep, sugar balance, immune function, and the proper hormonal balance during pregnancy.

✻ Hypothalamus—The Queen

The hypo in the name of this gland does not allude to hypo-function, but rather to its position in the brain. The hypothalamus is not a discrete structure but is part of the brain located under the thalamus, to which it is heavily connected with nerves. It is located deep within the brain, behind the eyes at the base of the optic nerves, and it is firmly attached to the pituitary via a stalk-like structure. The hypothalamus listens to all the feedback from the body that has to do with internal well-being, and it uses this information to release or inhibit the secretion of hormones produced by the pituitary. The Queen of the Hormones doesn't interact directly with her various endocrine gland subjects. Instead, she directs the King (the pituitary) to do the work. (As you can see, it's been scientifically proven that that's what men are for—to do the heavy lifting!)

Nerve transmissions and chemical messengers communicate directly with the pituitary to control a myriad of essential life functions that we don't even give a second thought to. Important life functions such as heart rate, blood pressure, breathing, body temperature, fluid balance, and directing all the other endocrine glands are all controlled by the hypothalamus. The hormones released by the hypothalamus are called releasing hormones and inhibiting hormones; as mentioned above, they directly influence the pituitary (more specifically, the anterior pituitary). In other words, a hypothalamic hormone will be secreted into veins that communicate between the hypothalamus and anterior pituitary and attach to the appropriate hormone receptor sites. The message sent to the anterior pituitary tells it which particular hormone is needed, and how much of it must be released or inhibited to create a certain necessary action in the body.

As an example, gonadotropin-releasing hormone (GnRH) from the hypothalamus binds to specific receptors on the anterior pituitary and causes stimulation of follicular-stimulating hormone (FSH). FSH is secreted directly into the blood and locates its target organs—the ovaries. GnRH also stimulates luteinizing hormone (LH) at a later time in the menstrual cycle. We discuss these activities further when we talk about the ovaries in more detail.

Figure 3.1 (on the following page) is a chart that demonstrates this three-part process of hypothalamus to pituitary to body part.

Figure 3.1

Hypothalamic Hormones	Anterior Pituitary Hormones	Tissue Affected
Thyrotropin-releasing hormone (TRH)	Thyroid-stimulating hormone (TSH)	Thyroid
Thyrotropin-releasing hormone (TRH)	Prolactin (PRL)	Breast
Gonadotropin-releasing hormone (GnRH)	Follicular-stimulating hormone (FSH)	Ovary
	Luteinizing hormone (LH)	Ovary
Growth hormone–releasing hormone (GHRH)	Growth hormone (GH)	All
Corticotropin-releasing hormone (CRH)	Adrenocorticotropic hormone (ACTH)	Adrenal
Somatostatin		Inhibits the release of growth hormone (GH)
Somatostatin		Inhibits the release of thyroid-stimulating hormone (TSH)
Dopamine		Inhibits the release of prolactin (PRL)

Hypothalamic Hormones	Posterior Pituitary Hormones	Tissue Affected
Antidiuretic hormone (ADH)	ADH is released	Kidney
Oxytocin	Oxytocin is released	Ovary

⚶ Pituitary—The King

The pituitary is often called the master gland, because it directly controls all the other endocrine glands. But, as we have seen, the power behind the throne is the hypothalamus. The King (the pituitary) waits for a message from the Queen (the hypothalamus) before going to work. Considering the important job that the pituitary has, it's surprising that it is only about the size of a pea and is located just behind the nose in an area scooped out of bone. The gland is composed of two main lobes, the anterior and posterior pituitary. Each performs different functions, as shown in the chart in Figure 3.2.

Figure 3.2

Anterior Pituitary

Hormone	*Tissue Affected*	*Effects Produced*
Growth hormone	Liver, adipose tissue	Protein, lipid, and carbohydrate metabolism
Thyroid-stimulating hormone	Thyroid gland	Stimulates secretion of thyroid hormones: T1, T2, T3, T4
Adrenocorticotropic hormone	Adrenal gland (cortex)	Stimulates secretion of glucocorticoids
Prolactin	Breast tissue	Milk production
Luteinizing hormone	Ovary and testis	Control of reproductive function
Follicle-stimulating hormone	Ovary and testis	Control of reproductive function

Posterior Pituitary

Hormone	*Tissue Affected*	*Effects Produced*
Antidiuretic hormone	Kidney	Conservation of body water
Oxytocin	Ovary and testis	Stimulates milk ejection and uterine contractions

Pituitary Malfunction

The pituitary rarely malfunctions, but when it does the most common disruptions that can occur include tumors, blood clots, and infectious diseases. After learning the various conditions that can arise from a damaged pituitary, mentioned below, you will understand the overwhelming importance of the pituitary in our lives.

Dwarfism: Deficiency of anterior pituitary hormones during childhood.

Acromicria: A condition that occurs after puberty where damage to the anterior pituitary makes the bones of the extremities small and delicate.

Simmonds's disease: Occurs in adulthood when extensive damage to the anterior pituitary causes premature aging, loss of hair and teeth, anemia, and emaciation; this is often a fatal condition.

Fröhlich's syndrome: A widespread disorder with an anterior pituitary deficiency and a lesion of the posterior pituitary or hypothalamus. The result is obesity, dwarfism, retarded sexual development, and dysfunction of the anterior pituitary hormones.

Acromegaly: Oversecretion of an anterior pituitary hormone, somatotropin, results in a progressive chronic disease characterized by enlargement of some parts of the body.

Diabetes insipidus: Deficiency of ADH from the posterior pituitary.

✎ Thyroid—The Princess

As I mentioned earlier, when I was in medical school the thyroid got most of the attention in endocrinology class. I call the thyroid "the princess" here because it's a misunderstood organ and women seem much more affected by thyroid problems than men. I have a special interest in the thyroid because my mother, after a hysterectomy for heavy uterine bleeding, was later diagnosed with hypothyroidism. Her doctor had thought she was just anemic and fatigued from years of heavy menstrual bleeding, and he didn't diagnose her hypothyroidism until she was almost lifeless. Many years later, when I became aware of the importance of the thyroid, I realized that her hypothyroidism may have caused her heavy bleeding and that she had been suffering from this condition for many years.

The thyroid is located on either side of and behind the windpipe. That's where doctors examine you to see if you have an enlarged thyroid, a condition called a goiter. Goiters form when there is a lack of iodine, and so they used to be a major clue to iodine deficiency. Now that iodine is added to salt, goiters are much less common. If you avoid salt for health reasons (or if you use non-iodized salts such as sea salt), you should make a special effort to get your daily supply of iodine, such as by eating more sea vegetables like kelp, nori, and kombu.

With its responsibility for the metabolism and temperature in all the body's cells, the thyroid literally runs the body. It's the motor in the engine. When there is too much thyroid hormone, the heart beats faster; when there's not enough, the heart and every other tissue and organ in the body slows down.

One of the thyroid's lesser-known functions is the stimulation of growth hormone, which is necessary for proper growth in infants. A thyroid deficiency in utero and in infancy can lead to brain impairment and mental retardation. Another little-known function is the secretion of a special hormone called calcitonin, which serves as the regulator of calcium in bones and blood. When the thyroid perceives a low amount of calcium in the blood, it secretes calcitonin into the blood, which triggers a release of calcium from the bones to bring blood calcium up to normal. When there is enough calcium in the blood, calcitonin is not secreted, and excess calcium (any amount above the normal blood levels) is transported into bone. The parathyroid glands, which we discuss later, have their own relationship with calcium.

Testing for Hypothyroidism

In his 1976 book *Hypothyroidism: The Unsuspected Illness*, Dr. Broda Barnes states, "Health begins and ends with the proper balance of the endocrine system." This is not far from the truth.

Dr. Barnes studied the thyroid all his life, and he maintained that the key to health was in balancing the whole endocrine system. About the thyroid, he said that the conventional thyroid function blood tests left many patients with clinical symptoms of hypothyroidism undiagnosed and untreated. If the blood test didn't indicate hypothyroidism, the patient was declared normal.

Knowing that the thyroid regulates the metabolic furnace of the body and controls temperature, Dr. Barnes told patients to take their morning temperature for ten days in a row. He advised menstruating women to begin taking their underarm temperature on the third day of their cycle. Specifically, when you wake up in the morning, stay in bed and place the thermometer under your arm. Going to the bathroom or even shaking down the thermometer before using it can elevate your temperature, so you should avoid doing either.

Another option is a basal thermometer, which some women use for fertility charting. It is more accurate and easier to read than a regular oral thermometer. (Please use a non-mercury thermometer to help curb the use of this dangerous metal.) Digital thermometers may not measure to the tenth of a degree that you want for the purpose of testing your thyroid.

Using your temperature, clinical signs, and the symptoms you mark on a questionnaire, along with blood tests, can give a more accurate picture of thyroid status than blood tests alone. Dr. Barnes was also convinced that patients who required thyroid replacement therapy received much more benefit from taking natural desiccated thyroid hormone than from taking synthetic thyroid hormones. Unfortunately, his work was not taught in medical school at the time I was there; we were told to rely on blood testing and use synthetic hormones. However, many doctors are now witnessing an epidemic in thyroid symptoms and educated patients are demanding desiccated thyroid therapy, all of which is changing the way hypothyroidism is being managed.

The following thyroid questionnaire will help you assess your thyroid function.

Place a checkmark next to any of the following signs or symptoms that you currently have.

- ❏ Fatigue
- ❏ Low body temperature
- ❏ Heart palpitations
- ❏ Poor concentration
- ❏ Memory loss
- ❏ Lack of motivation
- ❏ Difficulty sleeping
- ❏ Excessive need for sleep
- ❏ Trouble getting up in the morning
- ❏ Weak muscles
- ❏ Sore muscles
- ❏ Anxiety
- ❏ Panic attacks
- ❏ Depression
- ❏ Dry skin
- ❏ Itchy skin
- ❏ Unusual hair loss
- ❏ Dry hair
- ❏ Loss of outer third of the eyebrows
- ❏ Brittle or cracking nails
- ❏ Infrequent bowel movements or hard stools
- ❏ Constipation
- ❏ Gain weight too easily
- ❏ Persistent pain or swelling at the front of the neck
- ❏ Hoarseness
- ❏ Sensation of a lump in the throat
- ❏ Eye pain or double vision
- ❏ Swelling or protrusion of eyes
- ❏ Dry eyes
- ❏ Increased sweating
- ❏ Can't tolerate the cold
- ❏ Hand tremor
- ❏ Fluid retention
- ❏ Headaches, migraines
- ❏ Dizziness or lightheadedness
- ❏ Frequent colds or sore throats
- ❏ Skin infections, acne
- ❏ Rough skin
- ❏ Slow healing
- ❏ Slow speech
- ❏ PMS
- ❏ Menstrual problems
- ❏ Low libido
- ❏ Infertility
- ❏ Low blood pressure
- ❏ Elevated cholesterol
- ❏ Irregular periods
- ❏ Excessive menstrual flow
- ❏ Weaker menstrual flow
- ❏ History of miscarriage

Add up your checkmarks. Answering yes to as many as ten of the fifty symptoms is an indication of low thyroid. Take your temperature, as described above, and find a doctor that will take your clinical symptoms, your temperature, and your blood tests into account and also run a thorough panel of thyroid blood tests. If you do have low thyroid, ask for a hormone replacement called Armour Thyroid before taking synthetic thyroid. Armour Thyroid is a full thyroid replacement and not just the incomplete synthetic T4 found in most thyroid replacement drugs.

Hashimoto's Thyroiditis

You might never have even heard of it, but Hashimoto's thyroiditis is the most likely way a person becomes hypothyroid. It's classified as an autoimmune disorder, where antibodies attack the thyroid gland. The cause of Hashimoto's thyroiditis is said to be unknown. However, in a 2002 lecture, a neurosurgeon named Russell Blaylock made a point that I will never forget. He said that the word "autoimmune" implies that we are setting up an immune reaction to ourselves. But that is not the case: We are not attacking ourselves if we have a healthy body, but we can set up an immune reaction to an "abnormal self" riddled with inflammation and toxins, and with antigen/antibody reactions to these toxins and inflammatory products. Therefore, we may find in the near future that thyroiditis is a reaction to a toxic thyroid gland. We already know that various chemicals— namely malathion, which is used against West Nile virus—can cause thyroid damage and possibly lead to Hashimoto's thyroiditis.

The symptoms of Hashimoto's thyroiditis are very much like those for hypothyroidism: enlarged thyroid gland, fatigue, weight gain, and muscle weakness. However, one finding unique to Hashimoto's is that blood tests for thyroid antibodies are usually very high. After a period of months (or years) the thyroiditis calms down and the antibody levels fall, leaving a condition of hypothyroid. There is no medical treatment for thyroiditis, but various safe detox methods (which are discussed in Chapter 7) may help. When thyroid hormone levels drop due to the damage caused by the thyroiditis, thyroid replacement therapy is usually started. However, if the thyroid antibodies are still elevated, taking natural thyroid medications may cause the antibodies to attack the natural thyroid. People with elevated thyroid antibodies usually take synthetic thyroid replacement. In these cases, both T3 and T4 medications should be investigated instead of just settling for a T4 medication alone.

Hyperthyroid

As mentioned above, if there is too much thyroid hormone, the heart beats faster. And that's one of the main signs of hyperthyroidism. It's a condition that occurs when there is too much thyroid hormone acting on the tissues of the body. Symptoms of hyperthyroidism mostly have to do with a revved-up metabolism, and they include:

- Feeling hot and/or heat intolerance
- Weight loss
- Increased appetite
- Fatigue, especially at the end of the day
- Trouble sleeping
- Trembling hands
- Forceful and fast heartbeat
- Palpitations
- Increased bowel movements
- Irritability
- Nervousness
- Hair loss
- Shortness of breath
- Chest pain
- Muscle weakness

✤ Parathyroids

These four little-known glands—there are two attached to each side of the thyroid—are responsible for calcium and phosphate balance in the body. They mainly go awry when they are sometimes disrupted during thyroid surgery. They produce a hormone called parathyroid hormone, which helps build strong bones and keeps the heart muscle beating in tune to an electrical rhythm set by calcium. If your parathyroids have been removed during thyroid surgery, you must take calcium supplements along with magnesium and other bone-promoting nutrients. (We'll talk more about bone health in Chapter 10.)

✤ Adrenals—The Prince

The overt action and aggressiveness characteristic of the adrenal glands is what leads me to name them "the Prince." The adrenals are extremely important to our hormonal balance; Chapter 5 will be devoted to the role of the stress hormones, which are produced in the adrenal glands. Briefly, the adrenal glands sit on top of the kidneys. There are two of them and each only weighs about four grams—the size of an ordinary teaspoon. However, packed within that tiny teaspoon is a time bomb that we must learn to defuse. There are two parts to the adrenal gland, the medulla (the inside) and the cortex (the outside).

I was told in medical school that the adrenal medulla is not essential to life, but that when it is not working optimally it feels as if the life is draining out of you. It produces the hormones adrenaline and noradrenaline that cope with stress. Specifically, adrenaline increases the heart rate and the strength of heart contractions, increases blood flow to the muscles and brain, relaxes smooth muscles, and helps convert stored glycogen to glucose in the liver. Noradrenaline also increases blood pressure.

✖ Ovaries—The Twins

You can't have a hormone family unless you include the kids. Calling them "the twins" obviously makes sense because we have two ovaries, but it is also a tongue-in-cheek reference to the rise in the use of fertility drugs and the booming business of creating twins.

Balanced on the end of a curving fallopian tube, an egg-forming ovary sits on either side of the uterus. In an orchestration that also involves the hypothalamus and pituitary, the ovaries not only generate at least one egg once a month, but also produce estrogen and progesterone to create menstruation, pregnancy, and female sexual characteristics.

How the Ovaries Work

From about age twelve or fourteen—though usually occurring earlier in recent decades—the egg-producing activity of the ovaries is stimulated by FSH from the pituitary, which has been spurred into activity by gonadotropin hormone from the hypothalamus. Like clockwork each month (ideally, following the moon cycle), an egg develops inside a fluid-filled sac for nourishment. It's called a follicle—or from an ultrasound technician's point of view, a cyst.

The sac is nourishing a developing egg, which has another job of making and releasing estrogen. That estrogen helps build up the lining of the uterus (the endometrium) for a possible pregnancy. At a certain blood level of estrogen, the hypothalamus signals the pituitary to begin secreting another hormone involved with our menstrual cycle. It's called luteinizing hormone (LH). Through a wonderful feedback system, the rise in LH alerts the pituitary to reduce the production of FSH. Between day nine and day fourteen, the LH level peaks and the egg, which has inched its way to the edge of the ovary, takes the big leap. It pops out of the follicular sac, hopefully into the fallopian tube.

With the egg leaping about and preparing for its journey to meet the sperm in the uterus, the follicular sac now fills up with cholesterol and changes its name to the corpus luteum ("yellow body"). Progesterone is now made in abundance from this cholesterol—a very important substance that has been getting a bad rap from dieters (more on cholesterol in Chapter 4). During the first half of the menstrual cycle (called the follicular phase), estrogen has built up copious networks of blood vessels in the lining of the uterus. Now in the second half of the cycle (called the luteal phase), it's the job of progesterone to saturate the uterine lining with mucus and nutrients. You've probably guessed the rest: During the many months where the egg searches in vain for a sperm, the lining is sloughed off around day 28. The hormones come to a screeching halt and drop dramatically, which brings on the period.

Sacs Can Become Cysts

You might wonder what happens to all those sacs that form every month. We now know from ultrasound studies that a woman can have tiny 1- to 2-centimeter cysts in the ovary. In some cases the sac does not reabsorb. In an especially dramatic—not to mention gross—instance, a friend of mine had a sac the size of a football. It was aspirated by a long needle through the skin and produced a quart of fluid.

The Ovaries at Menopause

Our ovaries are responsible for the hormones that create our menstrual cycle, but they also produce hormones beyond our reproductive years—sometimes for decades after. From about age thirty-five, the outer covering of the ovary gets smaller and fewer eggs are formed. Around the time that a woman is in her mid-forties, something very interesting happens: The inner part of the ovary develops a life of its own and produces estradiol, progesterone, and androgens (male hormones) independent of follicles or corpus luteum cysts.

In other words, the ovaries stop producing eggs but not hormones! Dr. Christiane Northrup has reported this research for years in her newsletter and online writings. We therefore have three sources of hormones at menopause—hormones produced inside the ovary, hormones from the adrenals, and also hormones converted by the liver and kidney. Together they are important in the prevention of osteoporosis and the maintenance of libido. By taking good care of all these organs we can ensure enough hormones for our old age! We'll discuss this more in Chapter 7.

✖ Pancreas—The Insulin Behind the Throne

The pancreas produces digestive enzymes, but it is also responsible for secreting the hormone insulin, the prime regulator of blood sugar. Unfortunately, we usually only hear about insulin when someone becomes diabetic and must go on insulin shots. This is all too common, as the pancreas is under tremendous pressure in our sugar-coated, junk-food-craving society. Let's look at how insulin works to see why.

Insulin is secreted by the pancreas when the blood sugar rises. Its target is an insulin receptor site on all cell membranes in the body. When insulin reaches its goal it flips a switch that opens up the cell membrane to allow an influx of glucose, a cell's source of fuel. When someone eats processed foods or high amounts of sugar several times a day, the pancreas is programmed to react with a release of insulin to keep the blood sugar levels from going too high in the blood. If the pancreas didn't do this, the high blood levels of sugar created would be the equivalent of diabetes and could do damage to the eyes, kidneys, heart, and many other tissues and organs in the body. Just to put things into perspective, the blood usually has the equivalent of one teaspoon of glucose in the entire body at any one time, and yet when we drink a can of soda we supercharge our bodies with about ten teaspoons of sugar. It's like dynamite!

What's Bad about Insulin?

Pasta, sandwiches, and bagels, as well as sodas, all trigger a surge of insulin. High insulin forces glucose out of the bloodstream and into the cells. All of a sudden, your blood sugar is low, which makes you feel like you're starving, and you eat again—even if you just ate an hour ago. And so the vicious cycle goes. Before long, higher and higher amounts of insulin are needed to open up the cells of the body to receive glucose. The worst part is that high insulin shuts down fat burning, which is a disaster for someone who wants to lose weight. Diabetes means high glucose and high insulin levels. However, the medical treatment for diabetes is to give medications to force more insulin into the blood; this can cause even more weight gain. In Chapter 11, we discuss what makes a balanced diet and talk about how to keep your insulin levels balanced as well.

Insulin Resistance

After years of overworking the pancreas and chronically rising insulin levels by ingesting sixty teaspoons of sugar a day (the national average), there comes a time when the cells of the body no longer respond to the advances of insulin and they refuse the entry of glucose. The term for this condition is insulin resistance. When this sorry day comes, blood glucose levels rise and the body produces more and more insulin but nothing happens—the blood glucose stays high.

Abnormally high amounts of glucose and insulin saturate the body. This causes tissue damage that results in adult-onset diabetes, an increased risk of heart disease, and (as I learned when I wrote an earlier book on magnesium) magnesium deficiency. When magnesium is low it adds an extra burden to the heart and nervous system; makes cell membranes even more unresponsive to insulin; and impairs the 350 enzymes that depend on it. It's another vicious cycle. The key to health and longevity is keeping the blood sugar levels within a narrow range—not too high to trigger insulin, and not too low to trigger adrenaline.

Syndrome X

Syndrome X is newly invented medical term that seems to describe the effects of insulin resistance. Unfortunately, giving this condition a name distances this "new disease" from its origins— namely, a poor diet resulting in overstimulation of the pancreas and overworked insulin; a lack of the proper nutrients that are needed for metabolism such as the B vitamins, which leads to high homocysteine levels that damage the heart; and a lack of magnesium that can have health-threatening consequences.

The list of symptoms associated with Syndrome X includes hypertension, obesity, high cholesterol, elevated triglycerides, and elevated uric acid; it can lead to diabetes, angina, and heart attack. Dr. Gerald Reaven, who coined the term, feels that Syndrome X may be responsible for a large percentage of the heart and artery disease that occurs today.

Symptoms of Insulin Resistance

Scanning the symptoms of low thyroid (on page 51), which are similar to those of adrenal insufficiency (on page 93), some of the same symptoms appear with insulin resistance. This serves to show how interconnected the various endocrine organs are; when any one of them is sluggish, then the others react.

- Fatigue
- Poor concentration

- Bloating—excess digestive gas
- Sleepiness after a meal that contains even a moderate amount of carbohydrates
- Increased triglycerides
- Increased blood pressure

✳ Pineal

The pineal gland, located in the center of the brain above and behind the eyes, is about the size of a pea. It is able to measure day/night, light/dark cycles and release the hormone melatonin in response. The pineal, according to the *Encyclopedia Britannica*, "may play a significant role in sexual maturation, circadian rhythm and sleep induction, and seasonal affective disorder and depression. In animals it is known to play a major role in sexual development, hibernation and seasonal breeding."

Melatonin is produced in the body from the amino acid tryptophan. That's the key element in turkey that makes us all nod off after a big holiday meal. It is synthesized and released from the pineal gland when stimulated by darkness, with peak levels occurring early in the morning. Light inhibits the production of the hormone. Melatonin appears to have a role to play in regulating the ovarian-stimulating luteinizing hormone and follicle-stimulating hormone. It also regulates sleeping cycles, with more being produced at night. Research shows that using melatonin as a supplement can induce drowsiness.

✳ Brain Hormones

To make the overview of the endocrine system complete, I can't forget to mention the hormones that are produced in the brain; these are called *endorphins* or *enkephalins*. I received a special education in the importance of these hormones when I studied acupuncture. Apart from acupuncture working through the meridian system and thousands of acupuncture points, we have found in Western medicine that acupuncture increases the amount of endorphins in the blood and cerebrospinal fluid. A similar increase of these hormones occurs after a chiropractic spinal adjustment.

When the body is in pain or undergoing intense physical exertion, including sex, endorphins are produced. They are natural painkillers, much like opiates, produced in the hypothalamus that bind to receptors in the brain for pain relief. You have probably heard of the "runner's high"—well, it's really an "endorphin high." It helps to block the pain of the final mile in long-distance running. It also is responsible for the short-term loss of pain due to severe injury. It's the addiction to the "endorphin high" that may propel thrill seekers to engage in sky-diving, bungee jumping, and other extreme sports. Endorphins, as defined by Dr. Candace Pert, are the body's own morphine.

In 1992, Dr. Pert wrote her book *The Molecules of Emotions*, in which she discussed her discovery of opiate receptors. It wasn't until three years after her amazing research that a team in Scotland isolated the opiate produced by the body that fit into that receptor. They called it enkephalin, meaning from the head, whereas American researchers named their opiate endorphin, meaning endogenous morphine. The two terms are interchangeable, but endorphin is the one that is most used. We talk more about endorphins and stress in Chapter 5.

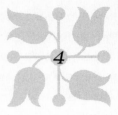

The Usual Suspects:
Estrogen, Progesterone, and Testosterone

WITH SO MANY MILLIONS of women taking synthetic estrogen and progesterone—and even testosterone—we have lost sight of the workings of the hormones that we make naturally in our bodies. An overview of the three main sex hormones will help us understand their roles in the body. In Chapter 13, we'll discuss their synthetic counterparts, and also their bioidentical twins.

The Origin of Hormones

Most people are surprised to learn that the female hormones (estrogen and progesterone) and the male hormone (testosterone) are all produced from the same molecule, and that this molecule is cholesterol. Cholesterol has become the bad guy in heart disease, but if we didn't have cholesterol we would all be in hormonal imbalance. In fact, it would be great to see some substantial studies done on people who are taking cholesterol-lowering medications and see whether their hormone levels are affected by medication. The only one I have been able to find was done on a mere 114 premenopausal women undergoing coronary angiography for heart disease.[14]

The following hormonal pathway diagram (Figure 4.1) was a nightmare to learn in medical school. It's just so important that I had to include it here. It shows that cholesterol is the precursor to not only the sex hormones—progesterone, estrogen, and testosterone—but also the stress hormone, cortisol. These hormones are produced in different sites—cortisol in the adrenals; progesterone mostly in the ovaries and placenta; and estrogen mostly in the ovaries—but they all need cholesterol to even get to square one. Therefore, cholesterol is stored in the adrenal glands and ovaries where it is available for whenever it is need to be converted to essential hormones.

Figure 4.1

Hormone Pathways

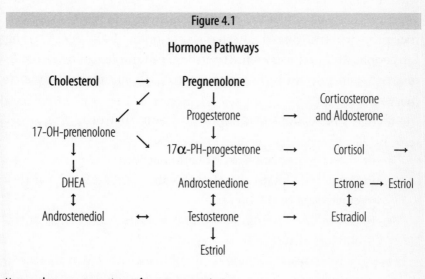

Note: ↓ = one-way action   ↕ = two-way action

✳ My History with Estrogen

My current views of HRT and ERT were molded in medical school. It was during my training, in the mid-1970s, that researchers finally had enough evidence to prove that taking estrogen pills promoted uterine cancer. The results created an immediate moratorium on estrogen use. My professors expressed concern about the drug and transferred that concern to their students. For example, we were told never to give estrogen to someone with cancer or a previous history of cancer. The same proscription holds today. I raised the obvious question: "How would I know if my patient had a subclinical undiagnosed cancer?" If I gave her estrogen I might be stimulating a microscopic cancer. How would I even know if one of my patients, in fact, had an early stage of cancer that I was unaware of, since we are presently unable to diagnose cancer until it has reached a state where it is visible to X-ray or palpation. If I gave my patient with subclinical cancer synthetic estrogen, would I be hastening her demise? That was one of the pivotal concerns in my career that further propelled me to learn alternative options and choices in caring for people, and that causes me to strongly promote wellness care in order to help prevent serious conditions such as cancer in the first place.

Here is a list of contraindications to using HRT or ERT:

- Previous cancer of breast or endometrium
- Precancerous lesions combined with a strong family history of carcinoma of the breast
- Breast-biopsy findings of precancerous lesions, such as ductal proliferation and cellular atypia
- Abnormal mammography findings: increased density, asymmetrical density, prominent ductal pattern, diffuse calcifications
- A strong family history of breast cancer in mother and sister (increases incidence four times)
- Severe fibrocystic disease of the breast
- Late first pregnancy
- Early menses onset and late menopause

The list of contraindications to HRT and ERT, in my mind, covers most of the female population. At last count, as many as one in two to three women are developing cancer; many women are postponing pregnancy; fibrocystic breast disease is becoming more common; and puberty is occurring in younger and younger children.

First Do No Harm

The dictate that physicians should "First Do No Harm" has always held real meaning for me, and I was not prepared to go against that principle with a known carcinogen. As time went on and the incidence of cancer rose, I became even more concerned about using estrogen, as I realized that a portion of that rise was due to estrogen use. Even when the pharmaceutical companies began promoting synthetic progesterone in an attempt to curb the estrogen-induced endometrial hyperplasia that led to cancer, I began to think this way: If one hormone (estrogen) shows such negative effects, how can adding another one (synthetic progesterone) make those symptoms go away? One reason that I was able to avoid the normal practice of prescribing synthetic hormones was the fact that I had so many alternatives to offer my patients. In Chapters 11 and 12, we'll talk about hormone alternatives and the use of natural hormone cream for vaginal atrophy.

Estrogen as a Carcinogen

The government is also aware that estrogen causes cancer—and they aren't just paying lip service to the problem. From 1992 to 2000, the Department of Defense Congressionally Directed Medical Research Programs awarded $1.5 billion for research conducted under the direction of Ercole L. Cavalieri, D.Sc., the director of the Center for Environmental Toxicology at the University of Nebraska. Dr. Cavalieri's research is focused on how cancer tumors are initiated by estrogens and polycyclic aromatic hydrocarbons (PACs). (These PACs are a standard product of combustion from automobiles and airplanes, and some are present in charcoal-broiled hamburgers.) Dr. Cavalieri believes that estrogen may be the cause of many common forms of cancer, including breast, ovarian, colon, pancreatic, and endometrial cancers, as well as non-Hodgkin's lymphoma, leukemia, and melanoma.

✂ The Three Sisters—Estrone, Estradiol, and Estriol

It is somewhat confusing to try to understand the three forms of estrogen. We'll discuss conjugated estrogens, synthetic versus natural estrogens, and bioidentical estrogens in Chapter 13, but first let's give a brief description of estrone, estradiol, and estriol. There is a numeric naming of the three estrogens. The –one in the word estrone means one, the –di in estradiol means two, and the –tri in estriol means (as you can guess by now) three.

In general, estradiol is the most bioactive estrogen of the three, and it is the most dominant hormone in growing up. The primary site of production of estradiol and progesterone is the ovaries; estrone is produced in abdominal fat cells; and estriol is mostly generated in the placenta during pregnancy. Some estrogens are also produced by the adrenal glands, which also produce the brother hormone, testosterone, in amounts one tenth the of males.

Not all estrogens are created equal in their functions and in their health benefits and health risks. However, estradiol is the form of estrogen that is the most common and the strongest; it is responsible for most of the estrogen functions in a non-pregnancy state (estriol is more active in pregnancy) and a non-menopausal state (estrone is more active in menopause).

Estriol has been identified as the "weak" estrogen when it's compared with estradiol. For example, in terms of replacement therapy,

2 to 4 milligram of estriol is equal to 0.6 to 1.25 milligrams of estrogen or estrone, and is just as effective. We obtain most of our information about estriol from Europe, where this milder hormone is the estrogen of choice. Compared to estradiol, which breaks down to estrone when given orally, estriol does not break down and remains intact as it is excreted.

✖ Estriol—The Pregnancy Estrogen

Estriol is labeled E1—it's not the most common estrogen in the body on a daily basis, but it is the most important estrogen for fetal development. Estriol depends mostly on estrone and partly on estradiol for its creation. A healthy liver is essential for its conversion from estrone. The ovary may secrete a small amount of estriol. Estriol is called the pregnancy estrogen, because it is produced almost entirely during pregnancy, and of the three estrogens it is the only one produced in the normal human fetus.

In fact, it is the fetal-placental production of estriol that leads to the progressive rise of estriol in the mother's bloodstream. The estriol urine test is used as a measure of the viability of the fetus. If the levels of urinary estriol fall dramatically during pregnancy, it can mean the fetus is in trouble. At all other times, the amount of estriol in the blood is very low. The seeming safety of estriol during pregnancy and the results of animal studies indicate that this form of estrogen is less cancer-causing than estradiol and estrone.

Estriol in Europe

Estriol can also be called the European estrogen, as it has been used there for almost fifty years. Studies, mostly done in Europe, show that estriol therapy causes very little endometrial proliferation. A buildup in the endometrium is the reason estradiol is unsafe for women who have an intact uterus. The use of estriol vaginal cream is becoming increasingly popular for postmenopausal vaginal atrophy and urinary incontinence; it is obtained on prescription through compounding pharmacies. Because it is a weaker form of estrogen, is used in its natural (bioidentical) form, and is not a patent medicine, U.S. drug companies have virtually ignored estriol. The "weak" effect of estriol may be partly what keeps it from having side effects like estradiol. In Chapter 13, we'll talk about the research being done to make sure estriol is safe and effective.

Estradiol—The Powerhouse

Estradiol is the main estrogen secreted by the ovary. It can also be created in the adrenal glands and converted from steroid precursor hormones in fat tissue. For a woman entering menopause, adding weight by gaining a pound a year is actually recommended by herbalist Susun Weed to aid in the creation of estrogen in your new fat cells.[15] Unfortunately, for most women it is not just estrogen that is created or stored in fat, but also xenoestrogens and other toxins that make excess fat unhealthy. So it's best to detox and make sure the fats you are eating can be healthy precursors to your hormones.

As an aside, for overweight women the amount of toxins stored in fat cells makes dieting a nightmare. As the fat cells break down during a diet, they release stores of chemical toxins that flood the bloodstream and can make you feel quite ill. Many women say they feel so bad when on a diet that the possible weight loss is just not worth it.

Estradiol Through the Cycle

In women who are actively menstruating, the amount of estradiol secreted daily varies widely—between 70 and 500 micrograms.

(A reminder: One microgram is one millionth of a gram and one gram is between ¼ and ⅓ of a teaspoon.) When measuring estrogen in the blood, the normal levels of estradiol fluctuate throughout the menstrual cycle, triggering effects when they are high or low.

For example, during the first week of the menstrual cycle (which is measured from day one of your period), estradiol levels remain nearly constant. There is a huge surge in estrogen, which causes luteinizing hormone (LH) to peak, which in turn causes ovulation to occur. After helping out with ovulation, the level of estradiol drops for several days and then rises again when the corpus luteum is formed. Estradiol blood levels are used to determine fertility, amenorrhea, and precocious puberty in girls.

When researchers first began looking at the female hormones, they focused on estradiol. This was because it's the most prevalent and the most potent form of estrogen; by comparison, estriol is mainly present during pregnancy, and estrone is mainly converted from estradiol or from androstenedione produced in the adrenal cortex.

The Roles of Estradiol

The functions of estradiol include breast growth and the maturation of the reproductive membranes (the primary sexual characteristics) and the development of pubic hair and underarm hair (the secondary sexual characteristics). Estradiol is also responsible for maturation of the long bones. Estradiol is produced mainly by the ovaries, with secondary production by the adrenal glands and conversion of steroid precursors into estrogens in fat tissue.

Estradiol continues its monthly pace until pregnancy occurs; at that time, it gives over control of estrogen to estriol formed in the placenta and in the developing fetus. For the perimenopausal period, we are now finding that estradiol, on average, is actually increased, not lowered. But around the time of menopause, estradiol finally does decline.

✗ Estrone—The End Result of Estrogen

Estrone is not secreted directly by the ovary but is created by a conversion from the androgenic (male) hormone androstenedione or from estradiol. Androstenedione is created mostly in the adrenal cortex, but some is also produced in the ovary. Research indicates that estrone may be even more carcinogenic than estradiol.

Synthetic estrogen usually consists of estrone alone, combinations of estrone and estradiol, or estradiol alone. However, when synthetic estradiol is taken orally it is mostly converted in the small intestine into estrone. Therefore, the end result of all these oral estrogens is estrone.

Androstenedione, which is made in the adrenal cortex, is also converted into estrone. Estrone is the most common estrogen found in menopause and in women who have had their ovaries removed surgically. The current thinking is that estrone may be carcinogenic in women who get breast cancer where their breast cancer has not been triggered by HRT. In Chapter 13, we'll talk about using hormone assays to determine the various levels of the three types of estrogen; and in Chapters 11 and 12, we discuss how you can improve your chances of creating the more beneficial hormones naturally in your body.

✗ What Estrogen Does

Before puberty, girls have very low levels of estrogen. Then, at a particular time in a young girl's life, mostly determined by her weight and the amount of adipose (fat) tissue she has, estrogen begins to stimulate primary and secondary sexual characteristics. The signs of puberty include development of breasts, pubic hair, and underarm hair. Through a complex feedback system, the hypothalamus produces FSH, which stimulates the ovary to develop an egg. Estrogen released from the sac that is nurturing the developing egg stimulates the lining of the uterus in anticipation of a pregnancy. Then, hopefully, menstruation begins on a regular monthly cycle.

During the reproductive years, estrogen's main function is to stimulate the growth of the uterus, breasts, and ovaries. It has been a common observation that women don't get heart disease nearly as often as men until after menopause. After a close study of blood lipids, it appears that estrogen elevates levels of HDL, the "good" cholesterol.

Estrogen and Moods

According to Marie-Annette Brown, Ph.D., author of *When Your Body Gets the Blues*, your estrogen and serotonin (the feel-good brain chemical) are both elevated during the first two weeks of your menstrual cycle. Then, in a wicked turn of events, the levels of both estrogen and serotonin plummet about a week before your period, leaving you moody and irritable. Estrogen does appear to be associated with elevated serotonin, but other researchers find that low levels of progesterone are responsible for the PMS mood swings. Either way, the cause is hormone imbalance.

Estrogen also stimulates the nervous system toward an outward focus. This fact has probably got something to do with biology and that primitive urge to seek out a male sperm donor! It has also been noted that during the second half of the cycle, when estrogen levels are falling, women become more introverted. Again, that may just be biology talking, trying to get us to slow down and get that sperm to take root and hatch a baby. It's all about the biology!

My History with Progesterone

As mentioned in Chapter 1, I developed a great deal of experience in my medical practice using progesterone for severe PMS. However, back in the 1980s, the only form of progesterone that wasn't immediately broken down in the liver and rendered useless was in rectal suppository form. Rectal suppositories of progesterone were not readily accepted by most women—even those who were desperate to find a solution to the life-destroying symptoms of PMS. We're just not a society that likes to take medicine in that form. It is surprising how Dr. Katrina Dalton has not only managed to convince women in the U.K. to use progesterone suppositories, but has also developed a worldwide reputation for her work.

In the United States, all we managed to do was declare PMS a psychiatric disease in 2001 by placing it in the DSM-IV (American Psychiatric Association's Diagnostic and Statistical Manual of Mental Disorders, 4th edition). Fortunately, pharmacists found a way to make bioidentical progesterone in a micronized form that was not destroyed immediately by the liver. But first, let's find out more about progesterone and its actions on the body.

✂ What about Progesterone?

For most people, estrogen is synonymous with being a woman. Very often the other equally important hormone, progesterone, is left out of the picture. Progesterone is made by the empty follicular sac in the ovary in response to stimulation by luteinizing hormone (LH), and it rises rapidly in the second half of the menstrual cycle. Progesterone is necessary for the "ripening" of the uterus. Estrogen sets the stage by supplying abundant blood supply, and progesterone creates the mucus and brings the nutrients. Along with estriol, higher and higher levels of progesterone are produced during pregnancy in the growing placenta. These high levels of progesterone act as a natural birth control that shuts down monthly ovulation for the duration of the pregnancy. Progesterone is also produced in the adrenal glands and is stored in fat cells.

During the first half of the menstrual cycle, the levels of progesterone are actually quite low. In the second half of the cycle, they surge up to a high level, and they remain there until menstruation occurs. However, progesterone remains low if ovulation fails to occur. There is a name for this type of cycle—anovulatory—and they begin to occur more frequently in women around the age of thirty-five. They also occur in young girls when they first begin their periods and can result in irregular periods and heavy bleeding; for this reason, doctors often prescribe the BCP to regulate them.

Anovulatory cycles may be another factor in perimenopausal symptoms. Many people have the impression that estrogen gets lower in the perimenopausal years, but research shows that estrogen actually becomes elevated, whereas progesterone levels fall markedly. And you can see why this is true, if a cycle does not trigger an ovulation and therefore progesterone is not produced. By the time of menopause, when estrogen levels are reduced to half of those of a thirty-year-old woman, progesterone can be approaching zero.

What Progesterone Does

As mentioned earlier, in order for a hormone such as progesterone to work, it must travel through the bloodstream, find a progesterone receptor, and become attached to that receptor to turn itself on. One of the most important functions of progesterone is to dampen down or counteract the effects of estrogen. In Figure 4.2 (on the following page), we see the dance between estrogen and progesterone where estrogen is the growth enhancer and progesterone is required to keep it from growing out of control.

Figure 4.2

The Female Cycle

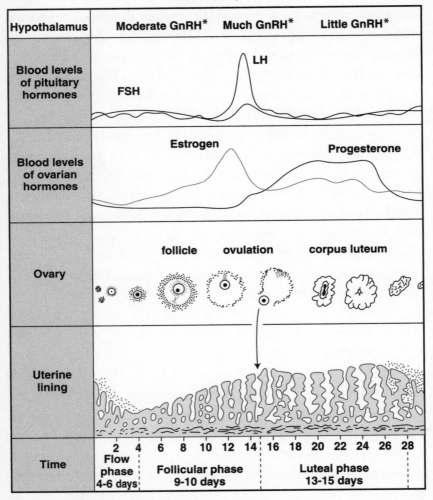

| Hypothalamus | Moderate GnRH* | Much GnRH* | Little GnRH* |

*GnRH means gonadotropin-releasing hormone.

As Figure 4.2 shows, progesterone's main job is to thicken the uterine lining with mucus and nutrients on its monthly quest for pregnancy. It also increases the sex drive, with the goal of making its job of preparing the uterus worthwhile! About 20 milligrams per day of progesterone is produced in what remains of the egg sac once it's left home to meet its mate. If the egg does not meet a suitable sperm that month, progesterone levels plummet, which causes the uterus to shed its lining and a period begins. If conception occurs, the placenta takes over the job of producing progesterone, to the tune of 400 milligrams per day.

Beyond preparation for pregnancy, progesterone has a multitude of effects throughout the body. You may know that estrogen is involved in bone production—well, so is progesterone. It also makes you sleepy and dampens anxiety, and it's involved in maturing the breast tissue and preparing the breasts for milk production. We have been able to tell a lot about what progesterone does by measuring the effects of an anovulatory cycle when progesterone is not produced in the second half of the menstrual cycle.

Progesterone Deficiency and Anovulation

Anovulatory cycles are one of the main reasons young girls are put on the pill. When the hormonal orchestration gears up in pre-teens and teens, it may be a little rough around the edges and it may take six to nine months to naturally sort itself out. As we saw with Zorra's story in Chapter 1, if children are unhealthy and underweight they might have trouble with their menstrual cycle. As we shall see in Chapter 6, xenoestrogens can also throw off the delicate balance of hormones operating in doses of one millionth or one trillionth of a gram. Sometimes six or nine months is too long for worried kids and anxious parents, who are used to quick fix solutions to all of life's problems, and for doctors, who think they have the solution in the form of the BCP. Anovulatory cycles keep progesterone from doing its part in the hormonal cycle and can cause:

- Irregular menstrual cycles
- Heavy menstrual bleeding

- Tender breasts
- Irritability and mood swings

Anovulatory cycles are also a common occurrence in women from their mid-thirties until menopause. At this phase of life doctors are likely to blame insufficiency of estrogen as the cause and may recommend HRT. When I was in medical school in the mid- and late seventies, we weren't taught anything about xenoestrogens. In fact, the research on this topic has only come out in the past two decades. I'm well aware of the fact that new "theories" have an incubation time of twenty to thirty years before they can break into the hallowed halls of science and medicine. In the meantime, we are unfortunately missing some of the true causes of hormonal imbalance.

Progesterone as Hormone Precursor

In Figure 4.1, if you follow the line from cholesterol to pregnenolone there is an arrow leading directly to progesterone that continues into the corticosteroids and cortisol pathway. We'll talk more about these adrenal hormones and stress in Chapter 5, but the message for now is that if progesterone becomes low, for whatever reason, our stress hormones suffer as well.

Comparing Estrogen and Progesterone

In the "what goes up must come down" world, the world of yin and yang, the play between opposites, estrogen and progesterone have opposite actions in the body and each is necessary to counterbalance the other. The following chart explains the actions of "unopposed" estrogen and the counter actions of progesterone.[16] Symptoms of excessive progesterone are rare; these might occur in pregnancy, or when a woman uses too much progesterone cream or takes too much natural oral progesterone. The side effects of synthetic progesterone (called progestins) will be dealt with in Chapter 13.

Figure 4.3

Comparing Estrogen Effects with Progesterone Effects

Estrogen	*Progesterone*
Creates uterine tissue lining for pregnancy	Creates and maintains mucus and nutrients in uterine lining for pregnancy (if no pregnancy, promotes shedding of the lining)
Causes breast tissue growth	Prevents fibrocystic breast disease
Promotes breast cancer by stimulating excess cell growth	Helps prevent breast cancer by opposing estrogenic growth activity
Promotes uterine cancer by building excessive uterine lining	Prevents uterine cancer by promoting shedding of uterine lining
Promotes ovarian cancer	Protects against ovarian cancer
Builds up uterine lining, increasing risk	Promotes shedding of uterine lining for endometriosis
Promotes depression and headaches	Acts as natural antidepressant
Interferes with thyroid hormone's ability to bind to cell receptor	Facilitates thyroid hormone cell binding to receptors
Stimulates excessive blood clotting	Balances blood-clotting activity
Leads to blood sugar imbalance	Balances blood sugar levels
Decreases sex drive	Increases sex drive
Produces body fat	Promotes the use of fat for energy
Promotes zinc depletion and copper excess	Balances zinc and copper levels
Causes minimal slowing of bone breakdown	Promotes bone building
Decreases vascular tone	Promotes normal vascular tone
Retains salt and fluid	Is a natural diuretic
Worsens PMS	Treats PMS
Increases insulin resistance	Prevents insulin resistance

✣ Estrogen Dominance

The main media message about estrogen is that it makes women feminine and fertile. When menopause occurs, estrogen loss is blamed. That's why it is so hard to convince the public—and many health professionals as well—that many of the health problems in our society may, in fact, be caused by too much estrogen and not enough progesterone. The term *estrogen dominance* was introduced by Dr. John Lee, an international authority and pioneer in the use of natural progesterone cream and natural hormone balance. In the early 1970s, Dr. Lee learned about the association between estrogen dominance and progesterone deficiency. From that time until his death in 2003, Dr. Lee worked avidly to educate the public and the medical profession about the need for more research on the subject of progesterone deficiency in the female population.

Knowing Estrogen Dominance

All through our lives we have felt estrogen dominance. It is the normal swelling of the breasts or tenderness of the nipples a few days before the period. It's when the breasts are swollen and tender for several more days in the month that you know your estrogen is high. Another sign of estrogen dominance is having heavy menstrual flow with clots and cramps along with irregular cycles. The timing of your periods may be every fourteen or seventeen days instead of every twenty-one, or you may be spotting all the time.

Estrogen Builds, Progesterone Breaks Down

In Chapter 2, I talked about the accumulation of research showing that estrogen given to women caused endometrial hyperplasia leading to uterine cancer. The medical answer to that problem was to add synthetic progesterone pills to the mix, creating HRT. The reason was that doctors know that natural progesterone, in the second half of the menstrual cycle, counters estrogen's buildup of new tissue and blood vessels and helps create the menstrual flow at the end of the cycle. When there isn't enough progesterone to stop estrogen, it can continue to build. Estrogen levels will taper off as production in the ovary naturally declines, but usually a considerable amount of endometrial tissue has built up, which creates a heavy menstrual flow. However, synthetic progestins cannot and do not act like natural progesterone.

What Causes Estrogen Dominance?

There are a variety of ways that a woman can be trapped by estrogen dominance:

1. The reliance on ERT for several decades before it was understood that it was causing uterine cancer caused millions of women to suffer symptoms of estrogen dominance.
2. Women who have had a hysterectomy are given just ERT because they don't have a uterus to overstimulate. However, this raises the question: What about all the other cells and tissues of the body that are suffering from estrogen dominance?
3. Presently, about ten million women are on ERT or HRT, both of which cause estrogen dominance. HRT consists of an estrogen component that causes estrogen dominance and a synthetic progestin that does not counter excess estrogen; it adds its own long list of side effects as well.
4. Young girls who are entering puberty, overweight, and exposed to xenoestrogens can have high levels of estrogen and experience painful periods. They are often given the BCP, which may stop their natural periods but keeps giving them daily hormones, increasing their estrogen dominance.
5. Estrogen dominance can occur during perimenopause,

when ovulation doesn't occur and there is little progesterone production in the last two weeks of the cycle.

6. Xenoestrogens (see Chapter 6) make the body believe that
   it has too much estrogen, causing estrogen dominance
   symptoms.

7. Another cause is when a poorly functioning liver is unable
   to manufacture the right balance of hormones from good
   cholesterol. In the movie *Super Size Me*, within a month of
   eating a McDonald's diet the filmmaker's liver enzymes were
   completely abnormal and his bad cholesterol and triglycerides were elevated.

8. A diet low in natural fiber can also contribute, as fiber helps
   bind and excrete excess estrogen.

9. Excessive alcohol use leads to liver damage and hormone
   imbalance. In one study, blood and urine estrogen levels
   increased up to 31.9 percent in women who consumed as
   little as two drinks a day.[17]

10. Birth control pills contain estrogen.

11. A hysterectomy (or tubal ligation) can cause dysfunction of
    the ovaries and create estrogen dominance.

12. Cortisol (the stress hormone) and progesterone compete for
    common receptors in the cells; cortisol impairs progester-
    one activity, setting the stage for estrogen dominance.

13. Postmenopausal women who are overweight and who have
    insulin resistance are candidates for estrogen dominance.

14. Another factor is obesity. Fat cells are a conversion site for
    estrogen.

The Symptoms of Estrogen Dominance

Estrogen dominance is not defined by a particular amount of
estrogen but by having too much estrogen relative to progesterone.
Estrogen can be all over the map—low, normal, or high—but if

there is little or no progesterone to balance its effects in the body, any amount of estrogen can create estrogen dominance. Thus the blood levels of estrogen can be "within normal limits" and the doctor will tell you "Your blood tests are normal, so everything is all right." But if he or she doesn't compare your estrogen levels with your progesterone levels, you might not find out that everything may not be all right.

Researchers say that estrogen is the hormone that makes women alert, focused, and extroverted (mostly in the first half of the cycle), but they don't remind us that progesterone creates calm and introversion. It's this balance in life as well as the balance in hormones that we are lacking. We don't need a hormone like estrogen to make us race around even more frenetically; we do need more calm and introversion by balancing our lives and hormones with progesterone.

Estrogen dominance has been noted by many prominent health professionals, such as hormone researcher Dr. Jerilynn Prior, gynecologist Dr. Christiane Northrup, and integrative medicine specialist and psychiatrist Dr. Serafina Corsello. It is common in the perimenopausal years, which in some women can begin around the age of thirty. Estrogen overstimulation affects all the tissues of the body. Here are some of the effects of estrogen without the balancing action of progesterone:

- Decreased sex drive (Progesterone is actually the "sexy hormone.")
- Irregular periods (Without progesterone, you have anovulatory cycles.)
- Heavy periods
- Bloating and fluid retention
- Breast swelling and tenderness (Estrogen promotes breast tissue growth.)
- Fibrocystic breasts
- Headaches (this can be part of the fluid retention)

- Mood swings
- Weight gain in the abdomen and hips
- Hair loss
- Thyroid abnormalities—cold hands and feet, sluggish metabolism, and fatigue
- Foggy thinking and memory loss. While just enough estrogen can make you alert, too much can do the opposite.
- Insomnia
- Fibroids are stimulated by estrogen and resolve at menopause
- PMS
- Infertility
- Cancer

Estrogen Dominance and Cancer

Cancer seems to be the defining disease in how we decide whether or not something is "really serious." When the incidence of endometrial cancer went from almost nonexistent in the female population to alarming rates after women started taking oral estrogen in the form of Premarin, the medical establishment took notice and stopped using it in women who had a uterus. The same cautions occurred after the Women's Health Initiative study. As soon as we could scientifically say that taking synthetic progestin does not protect a woman from the cancer-causing effects of synthetic estrogen, recommendations were made to drastically cut back its usage.

Now it seems we can say that estrogen causes cancer in many tissues of the body, and not just in women and not just in the sex organs and tissues. By exploring estrogen dominance and realizing its many causes noted above, it appears that we can draw at least a preliminary conclusion that estrogen and xenoestrogens may be partly responsible for the high incidence of cancer in our society.

Counting Breast Cancer

The incidence figures of cancer are staggering. According to the National Center for Health Statistics, the number of women who have breast cancer is about 131 per 100,000. Every year another 180,000 American women are diagnosed with breast cancer and 44,000 will die. A woman dies every twelve minutes of breast cancer in America. The World Health Organization reports that 1.2 million women worldwide will be diagnosed with breast cancer this year.

In 1996 the American Cancer Society published historical figures on the mortality rate of breast cancer. We might assume that compared to 1930 we would have a lower annual death rate because of increased medical technology. However, in 1930, when the only treatment was mastectomy, the death rate for breast cancer was 25 per 100,000 women. The 2002 death rate is almost 29 per 100,000. We have regressed, not progressed, in being able to save lives. The incidence of breast cancer has risen an average of 1 percent per year between 1940 and 1982. In the twenty-five years between 1973 and 1998, breast cancer incidence rose by 40 percent. Many environmentalists believe that various environmental factors are to blame. It was during the 1970s that we developed a love affair with chemicals and pharmaceuticals. We'll talk more about these sources of estrogens and xenoestrogens in Chapter 6.

✂ Talking to Progesterone

Perimenopause and menopause are affecting tens of millions of women, and this has produced a proliferation of information on the Internet. Much of this information is geared toward the use of progesterone cream to balance estrogen dominance. In theory, I agree with the concept, but in Chapter 13 I'll show reasons why women must be cautious about jumping on the progesterone cream bandwagon.

When you read information on Web sites selling progesterone cream, you will find health claims for progesterone that border on the incredible and even the miraculous. Part of the explanation for these claims of remarkable results is that progesterone is a precursor to the adrenal hormones, cortisol, and corticosteroids; to testosterone; and to DHEA. If you look at the chart in Figure 4.1 on page 63, you can follow the arrows that are connected to all these hormones. Therefore, all the symptoms of adrenal exhaustion—allergies, autoimmune disorders, hypoglycemia, and mood swings—may be affected. Even a thyroid that has been bound up with estrogen can be released by proper amounts of progesterone, thus leading to a lessening of thyroid symptoms.

Wow! you might say—even more reason to take progesterone cream and increase all your hormones! However, estrogen is also on the progesterone pathway, and while you may be increasing progesterone you are also pumping up your estrogen. You have to keep in mind that, as we've discussed before, hormones are active in infinitesimal quantities, and if you just slather on progesterone cream you may be promoting untoward side effects. By thinking that progesterone is the "cure," we fall into the same old pattern of seeking the magic bullet—there's more to a balanced life and balanced hormones than fighting back potentially high estrogen with progesterone cream. But don't worry, there really are safe ways to balance your hormones.

Testosterone

Men are identified with testosterone in the same way that women are with estrogen. But just to spice things up, each sex has a bit of the other's major hormone. Women make seven times less testosterone than men, and it's produced equally in the ovaries and adrenals. In men, there is little question about where it's made, as it all comes from the testicles.

When we see big, muscular men, we tend to think of lots of testosterone. In women, it doesn't go quite that far; however, studies in women do show that testosterone helps make muscles stronger and bones denser and also gives the sex drive a bit of a lift. Most blood and saliva panels to test for hormones include testosterone; if it is deficient, many women report that using small doses can improve their quality of life.

The reasons for deficiency of testosterone are varied. Total hysterectomy that removes the ovaries along with the uterus cuts the production of testosterone in half. Stress that burns out the adrenals can diminish production in those organs. ERT or HRT can suppress testosterone production in the ovaries by partially shutting down signals from the pituitary. The pituitary thinks there are enough hormones in the blood (even though they are synthetic) and doesn't push the ovaries to make any more.

Symptoms of testosterone deficiency include:

- Muscle weakness
- General weakness
- Lack of energy
- Lowered sex drive

The side effects of too much testosterone replacement therapy include:

- Acne
- Facial hair growth
- Male-pattern baldness

What about DHEA?

There is a lot of talk about DHEA, which is a weak male hormone. People are taking it as a supplement in hopes that it will prop up flagging hormones. However, there's a catch. If you remember the hormone diagram in Figure 4.1, you can see arrows going from DHEA to testosterone and also to estrogen. Supposedly, DHEA is converted to testosterone in men, and estrogen is made from DHEA in women. There is also a slight crossover effect, though, which means that men will get extra estrogen and women will get extra testosterone. If you are a woman with too much estrogen already, you might not benefit from taking DHEA at all. DHEA levels do drop as you get older, and research does show that taking the hormone can improve sexual function in women who already have low-functioning adrenal glands. We'll talk more about DHEA in Chapter 12.

5

Stress Hormones Tip the Balance

ARE YOU TIRED OF HEARING how everything is worsened by stress, and that stress causes every condition known to woman? I know I am. Actually it's even more frustrating, because in order to avoid stress you have to become another person. You have to stop working, stop worrying, stop eating, and stop getting bugged by things—all of which is only possible if you win the lottery or move to a desert island, each of which brings its own stresses! Stress has become the scapegoat for so much unwellness for a good reason, though. Maybe when you understand why, and also learn the specific nutrients that will treat stress, you won't be so stressed by stress.

It's All about Stress

You can't talk about stress without mentioning Dr. Hans Selye, the Canadian endocrinologist. Selye actually invented the term around 1936. It wasn't until 1950, though, that Dr. Selye published his magnum opus *Relief from Stress*, a weighty 1,000 pages with 5,000 references. His dedication in the front of the book gives some important evidence about the many diverse causes of stress. Having lived through two world wars, Dr. Selye found a special meaning in stress. His dedication reads:

> To those who—in their efforts for good or evil, for peace or war—have sustained wounds, loss of blood or exposure to extremes of temperature, hunger, fatigue, want of air, infections, poisons, or deadly rays.
>
> To those who are under the exhausting nervous strain of pursuing their idea—whatever it may be, to the martyrs who sacrifice themselves for others, as well as to those hounded by selfish ambition, fear, jealousy, and worst of all by hate.
>
> For my stress stems from the urge to help and not to judge.
>
> But most personally, this book is dedicated to my wife, who helped so much to write it, for she understood that I cannot, and should not, be cured of my stress but merely taught to enjoy it.

Selye's book dedication shows us that any and all emotions, any and all external toxins, and any and all physical needs can be interpreted by the body as stress. It gives us a far greater understanding of stress than a dictionary definition, which generalizes that stress is "mental, emotional, or physical strain caused, for example, by anxiety or overwork. It may cause such symptoms as raised blood pressure or depression."

But let's not forget that inherent in stress is often a chance to overcome that stress, learn from it, and become stronger. The closest Chinese word that signifies stress is depicted by two characters—the upper one is Danger, the lower one is Opportunity. Dr. Selye was able to prove that on a day-to-day basis we are affected by stress of two natures: pleasant stress that translates into "wellness" and unpleasant stress that translates into disease and sickness.

Dr. Richard Earle, co-founder, along with Dr. Hans Selye, of the Canadian Institute of Stress, says, "If you're alive you have no choice but to see your stress level go up hundreds of times a day. Think of your stress as the energy you invest in your life. From this viewpoint, 'good stress' is the experiences you have when you get lots of satisfaction back from the stress you spend. And, 'bad stress' shows up when your returns-on-investment are low, as in fatigue, frustration or getting the flu frequently."

The History of Stress

Born in 1907 into a long line of medical doctors, Selye entered the German Medical School in Prague at age seventeen. He graduated first in his class and went on to earn a doctorate in organic chemistry. As a medical student, he noted that there were identical symptoms and signs that patients experienced in spite of having different diseases. One of the many beliefs that made Dr. Selye unique was the way he questioned medicine for concentrating its efforts on labeling diseases and trying to find a drug to cure them "without giving any attention to the much more obvious 'syndrome of just being sick.'" Out of these observations he discovered "a group of signs and symptoms that occur together and characterize a disease." He called it the "General Adaptation Syndrome," the body's hormonal response to stress that leads to ulcers, high blood pressure, arteriosclerosis, arthritis, kidney disease, and allergic reactions. His first major publication describing his findings was "A Syndrome Produced by Diverse Nocuous Agents" published in 1936 in *Nature*. His concepts broke down boundaries in the various sciences because his work impacted biology, biochemistry, physiology, endocrinology, animal husbandry, sociology, and psychology.

General Adaptation Syndrome (GAS)

Stress is the nonspecific response that anyone exhibits to demands on the body. The demands could be very minimal, such as taking an energetic walk, doing homework, or planning an exciting vacation. It could be jumping out of the way of a bicycle or even tripping over your own feet. We gear up our own stress hormones when we psych ourselves up to give a speech or when hitting a personal snag in a relationship. Here are three stages that this response to stress can go through:

Alarm Phase

In Chapter 3, we discussed the alarm reaction. It's the fight-or-flight response that occurs when the body feels it is under attack and releases adrenaline in preparation for a battle or a swift run. It's actually a normal protective mechanism that has saved many lives. Blood surges to the heart and muscles, the heart beats faster, breathing increases, the eyes dilate, and the stomach tightens up.

Adaptation Phase

In this phase the body gets the message that it's dealing with long-term stress. The corticosteroid hormones that come into play here increase blood sugar levels to sustain energy and raise blood pressure. The adrenal cortex produces corticosteroids that are also called cortisol. We'll speak more later about cortisol and its role in causing disease when it is overproduced in the body. The symptoms of too much cortisol are fatigue, concentration lapses, irritability, and lethargy.

Exhaustion Phase

In this phase, not only is the body exhausted, so are the adrenal glands; the body and the adrenals have no reserves. The body, mind, and spirit are exhausted. The blood sugar levels decrease, causing symptoms of hypoglycemia. The immune system is also exhausted, leading to illness and collapse.

✎ Women and Stress

As with most scientific research, much of the early clinical stress research was performed on men. Over time the different responses of men and women to stress became more obvious. Stress makes men angry; they get mad and try to blame someone. They may boil like a cauldron and then periodically erupt like Vesuvius. The eruption process occurs internally, as well as in outbursts of anger and temper. Men develop ulcers, high blood pressure, and heart disease, and they may turn to alcohol as a pacifier or distraction.

Women tend to withdraw to their family, friends, or themselves when under stress. The conditions they develop are depression and anxiety. Women are diagnosed with more post-traumatic disorders and autoimmune diseases. Recent research at UCLA supports this tendency of women to withdraw inward. Women have higher levels of a hormone called oxytocin. It is a powerful mood balancer that is increased by the presence of estrogen but decreased in the presence of testosterone. Oxytocin creates a desire for social support and sharing, instead of the fight-or-flight response seen more often in men.

Dr. Richard Earle says that the different responses to stress may explain why "When lost on a trip, women will ask for directions while men don't, not wanting to feel weak and vulnerable doing so. It may also account, in part, for why women live seven years longer than men."

✎ It's All about the Adrenal Glands

The adrenal medulla produces the stress hormones of "alarm." However, too much "alarming" stress can deplete the adrenaline hormones. We all know about adrenaline, the fight-or-flight hormone. It floods out of the adrenal medulla into the bloodstream when we get a fright or a shock. Its job is to increase the heart rate and increase blood going to the heart and extremities. At the same time it shuts down the blood flow going to the stomach and intestines.

Adrenaline protects us by making more blood and oxygen available to our legs so we can run from danger, and providing more to our arms and legs in case we have to fight. You've probably heard of people getting an adrenaline shot for an attack of asthma. That's because adrenaline also opens up the air passages in the lungs so we can get more oxygen to transmit to the blood and on to our muscles. A slightly nasty side effect of adrenaline is that it stimulates the bowels and bladder to evacuate. That explains why a sudden shock or stress, like an upsetting phone call, always seems to give you the urge to go.

Looking at the mechanism of our physical, mental, and emotional reactions to stress helps us to understand how stress works; it can also give us tools to modify our stress. For example, during an alarm reaction when blood flows to the muscles and heart, there is a relative shutdown to the stomach and intestines. The stomach can tighten up into a fist and even lead to esophageal reflux, commonly called GERD (gastroesophageal reflux disorder). Shutting down blood flow to the stomach also can prevent the natural production of stomach acid, which leads to undigested food causing heartburn and bloating.

The adrenal cortex produces the corticosteroid hormone, called cortisol, during the adaptation phase of the stress response. Its main job is to try to "get along" with invaders and inhibit inflammation that they may produce. In the mildest sense this could be a calming reaction to pollens in the spring. If stress takes a more dangerous turn, cortisol is able to convert protein to energy, a very important function if all the glucose and glycogen stores have been used up in the alarm phase of a stress reaction. Cortisol also suppresses inflammation and strengthens the immune system. Cortisol is released continuously when you get only five or six hours of sleep, shrug off those drooping eyelids, and push yourself too hard. It's not meant to used as your "personal energizer," though. Cortisol is just a backup system, and it will eventually become depleted.

Another product of the adrenal cortex is aldosterone. It regulates sodium excretion in the urine to keep the blood pressure normalized. A third type of adrenal cortex hormone is the androgenic steroid that is related to male hormones.

✕ Signs of Adrenal Exhaustion

This "Personal Stress Checklist" comes from Dr. Richard Earle at the Canadian Institute of Stress. This checklist helps you recognize that the "anxiety" symptoms you may be having are really due to stress.

❏ Inability to concentrate	❏ Indigestion
❏ Pounding heart	❏ Queasy stomach
❏ Irritability	❏ Difficulty making decisions
❏ Erratic behavior	❏ Excessive worry
❏ Dry mouth and throat	❏ Brooding
❏ Restlessness	❏ Trembling
❏ Emotional tension	❏ Tics
❏ "Keyed-up" feeling	❏ Sudden increases in smoking or alcohol use
❏ Cold, clammy hands	
❏ Impulsive behavior	❏ Feelings of worthlessness
❏ Jumpiness	❏ More frequent illnesses
❏ Headaches	❏ Difficulty getting along with people
❏ Poor judgment	❏ Forgetfulness
❏ Frequent mistakes	❏ Insomnia
❏ Much daydreaming	❏ High blood pressure

✕ The Adrenals and Blood Sugar Stress

We'll be talking about the best diet to balance your hormones in Chapter 11, but as the adrenal glands are so intimately connected with the amount of sugar in our blood, and low blood sugar creates a major stress in the body, it's important to also talk about it here.

Juggling Donuts

Blood sugar, called glucose, is supposed to stay within a certain normal range and the body makes sure it does by an intricate system of feedback controls. If you eat a bagel with jam, a sugared donut, or toast with honey for breakfast, the simple carbohydrates of sugar and white flour are easily broken down into glucose and rapidly absorbed into the bloodstream, because there is no fiber to slow down that absorption. When a load of glucose hits the bloodstream, it rings off an alarm in the pancreas to release insulin, which has the job of opening up the body's cells to receive glucose.

One Teaspoon of Sugar in the Blood

There is no question that glucose is a necessary food for the body and the brain, but we normally only have about one teaspoon of sugar in our bloodstream at any one time. Yet, a can of soda has about ten teaspoons! When you ingest ten teaspoons of refined sugar from sugar cane and discard the fiber, or eat beet sugar without the fiber from the beets, the sugar hits the bloodstream like a sledgehammer. The sugar very quickly reaches an alarming level in the blood, and the pancreas is jolted into releasing an excessive amount of insulin to deal with the excess sugar. After all, when the body knows that one teaspoon is the maximum amount the bloodstream can handle, it goes into overdrive to get rid of the other nine teaspoons from the soda you just drank.

Insulin at Work

Insulin's job is to open up little doors in the cells of the body to receive glucose that the cells use to produce energy. If a great amount of insulin is released, a lot of cells open up to absorb the glucose and then the blood sugar can fall dramatically. One minute the blood sugar is too high and the next minute it's too low. Such a dramatic shift signals danger in the body.

Hypoglycemic Reaction

When the blood sugar crashes you can feel sweaty, woozy, dizzy, and headachy; all kinds of alarms go off, and your body goes on red alert. Your adrenal glands, which are located on top of your kidneys, respond to the alarm and flood your body with adrenaline. The same thing happens when you get a big fright, such as having a near-collision while driving or having a tremendous noise go off behind you. It's adrenaline that allows a mom to pick up the rear end of a car when her kid is trapped underneath. It's a survival mechanism called fight-or-flight. It also stimulates the sugar stores called glycogen in the liver to make sure the blood sugar stays stable. But there's a downside to adrenaline. With all that stimulant flooding the bloodstream—especially when all it has to do is take care of low blood sugar and you're not burning it off by running or fighting—you can get a feeling of anxiety, because your heart is pounding and you feel shaky and nervous.

That is why a coffee and a donut in the morning is the worst way to start your day. They may give you a quick jolt and get your eyes open, but it won't be long before you crash and then feel you need another hit of sugar. If you continue this cycle of soaring and crashing, your pancreas and adrenals are both going to suffer. Over time, the excess insulin causes the body's cells to shut the door on insulin. This is called "insulin resistance," which you read about in Chapter 3. Insulin resistance is the road to diabetes.

Living on Empty

The roller coaster of blood sugar is like a microcosm of the life many women live. The battle cry used to be "shop till you drop," but that's been replaced by "work till you drop." Families these days seem to need two incomes just to keep up. Women are working just as hard as men at work; and at home they are working even harder, as they put in much longer hours on meal preparation, child care, laundry, and home cleanup. I hear stories all the time from women clients who literally work until they drop. They put in ten-hour days at work and come home to another four or five before crashing into bed. They have no more reserves of energy left coming from their adrenal glands.

Unfortunately, insomnia is one of the effects of high output of adrenaline and cortisol. It's like you can't find the switch to turn yourself off. Your mind races, your heart races, your legs twitch as if you're running the four-minute mile, and you can't shut down. Insomnia further tears away at your dwindling reserves of energy. Some women are able to keep up this maddening pace by catching up on sleep over the weekend. More often than not, work has a way of forcing itself into that sacred space. As energy goes down productivity also goes down, so it's a constant game of catch-up. Most people haven't learned very much about nutrition and the brain's absolute requirement for certain nutrients. Instead of using essential fatty acids, B vitamins, and magnesium to boost their physical and mental energy, many people turn to coffee and sugar.

Uppers and Downers

Dr. Richard Earle talks about the three sets of hormones involved in the stress roller coaster. They are:

1. "Uppers" such as adrenaline, which rises dramatically when we get revved up to meet a demand.

2. "Modulators" such as noradrenaline, which allows us to stay very revved up (at high RPM) without too much risk of sudden cardiac death.

3. "Downers" such as cortisol, which our body—being a very wise mechanism—injects when it knows we've been revved too high for too long.

Dr. Earle says it's the cortisol "downers" that are responsible for us crashing after an impossibly hectic couple of weeks. That's the time to really listen to your body and take a much needed break and build up your reserves. Of course, you may not listen when your body gets bone-weary. You may chide yourself and push even harder to meet some deadline, or keep up with some level of energy or workload you think you should have. Coffee serves as a powerful drug to keep whipping your adrenal glands to release the hard stuff—the adrenaline "uppers" you need to keep up the pace. You have to really force the adrenaline out at this stage, because with cortisol in the body the adrenaline has to overcome its calming effect. Runners who get their high after several miles are doing the same thing to their adrenal glands, beating them harder and harder to get that rush.

ﾟ It's All about the Cortisol

Dr. Margaret Merrifield, and many other integrative medicine doctors, have been chanting this litany for years. In her filled-to-capacity woman's clinic, Dr. Merrifield has found that depleted adrenal glands set the stage for a host of problems, especially a difficult perimenopause and menopause. Since the adrenal cortex secretes both estrogens and androgens (male hormones—just think of those chin hairs!), and it becomes the primary site for progesterone production around the menopause, the adrenal glands must be supported.

Our need for adequate cortisol to deal with stress is just as important as our need for the adrenals to produce sex hormones. Treating the adrenal glands is Dr. Merrifield's first step to restoring hormonal and physical equilibrium in her patients. If there is unremitting stress or even low-grade but constant stress, the production of cortisol continues. The hypothalamus is wired to interpret the stressors in the environment and in our bodies and continues to signal the adrenals to deal with the stress.

Cortisol's Place in Stress

Chronic production of cortisol due to exposure to the above stressors leads to:

- Depletion of the adrenals, causing fatigue and depression
- Diminished production of mood-enhancing serotonin
- Suppression of the immune system through increased production of interleukin-6, an immune-system messenger, leading to effects from colds to cancer
- Fat and cholesterol accumulation in the arteries
- Connective tissue thinning
- Impaired cellular utilization of thyroid hormones
- Imbalance of the healthy circadian hormonal rhythms
- Disturbance of the healthy regulation of blood glucose
- Impaired insulin utilization
- Insomnia

"Impaired insulin utilization" in the list above may not sound that bad, but remember what we discussed in Chapter 3. Too much insulin causes carbohydrate cravings and can result in a lot of symptoms that you don't want, like weight gain and bloating.

✐ Stress and the Pause—Let Me Count the Ways

It's not enough to say everything causes stress (although it does). You need to remember that some stress is good and some is bad. Let's go over the list of possible negative stresses in your life so you can put them into perspective and hopefully on the back burner. So you won't get too stressed out by this list, one thing you should know is that physical exercise burns off the excess stress hormones that can flood your body.

Just having written this last sentence I got restless. I knew it was time to do some exercise, but I didn't want to do my usual yoga and I didn't feel like going for a walk. I absentmindedly went to check the mail while deciding what to do about the stress of inactivity. And there in my basket was a new set of exercise tapes called T-Tapp. I immediately put a DVD in my computer; I not only learned about my body type, but after fifteen minutes I felt as if I'd had a big workout. I'll talk more about T-Tapp in Chapter 11. Now, I really feel much more motivated to tackle this list of stressors, and my evil twin, who wanted me to stop writing, has been banished.

Internal Body Stressors

As Dr. Selye said in the dedication of his book *Relief from Stress*, stress can be from:

- *Sustained wounds:* Any injury, accidental or planned as in surgery.
- *Loss of blood:* Menstrual periods, surgery, or accidents.
- *Exposure to extremes of temperature:* Winter and summer both have their stresses from wearing clothing inappropriate for the weather.
- *Hunger:* Starvation diets, or the malnourishment of processed and junk foods.

- *Fatigue:* Especially for mothers: the results of sleep deprivation, overwork, and the strain of managing work and a family.
- *Want of air:* The pollution in the atmosphere that gives us less oxygen than we need for healthy metabolism.
- *Infections:* Even the simple flu can be deadly if our immune system is depleted due to stress, and chronic infections can trigger the release of stress hormones—another vicious cycle.
- *Poisons:* There are about 100,000 industrial chemicals in our environment, and dozens to hundreds of chemicals can be found in our cells and tissues.
- *Deadly rays:* X-rays may be a diagnostic life saver, but every X-ray has the potential to cause DNA damage.
- *Exhausting nervous strain* of pursuing an idea.
- *Martyrs* who sacrifice themselves for others.
- Those hounded by *selfish ambition, fear, jealousy,* and worst of all by *hate*.

In his book *Healing the Planet*, the clinical ecologist Dr. Jozef Krop, Fellow of the American Academy of Environmental Medicine, gives the following list of stressors:

CHEMICAL STRESSORS
- Organic substances such as formaldehyde, phenol, benzene, toluene, and xylene, plus many chemicals derived from gas, oil, and coal.
- Organic chlorinated compounds, including organochlorides, pesticides, chloroform, pentachlorophenols, polychlorinated biphenols (PCB), and various herbicides such as 2,4-D (2,4-dichlorophenoxyacetic), and other pesticides.
- Inorganic substances such as mercury, lead, cadmium, aluminum, asbestos, chlorine, nitrous oxide, sulfur dioxide, ozone, copper, nickel, illegal drugs, tobacco smoke, and medications.

PHYSICAL STRESSORS
- Heat, cold, weather cycles
- Noise
- Positive and negative ions
- Electromagnetic radiation (full range of the light spectrum)
- Ionizing radiation (radioactivity from X-ray, atomic explosions, reactor accidents, reactor leaks, food irradiation, radon gas)

BIOLOGICAL STRESSORS
- Bacteria
- Viruses
- Fungi (molds)
- Parasites
- Foods
- Animal dander
- Dust
- Pollens from trees, grasses, and weeds

PSYCHOLOGICAL STRESSORS
- Prolonged psychological stress in the family (alcoholism, sexual abuse, family disruption, prolonged sickness of a family member, etc.)
- Prolonged psychological stress at work (overwork, poor relationships, job loss, etc.)
- A death in the family
- Loss due to fire, bankruptcy, etc.

High Cortisol = No Weight Loss

That's right, when you are under stress and have high levels of cortisol, your body is physiologically unable to go into a weight-loss mode—it's that simple. Elevated stress hormones make the body believe that there is danger afoot. And in dangerous times you need to conserve all your fat reserves for the crises that the body perceives. The body is very smart and has good reason for everything it does. But sometimes we give it the wrong message—in this case, by not knowing how to turn off our stress.

Another reason why weight gain is becoming epidemic may be due to the fact that your body stores fat-soluble chemicals (pesticides, herbicides, and heavy metals) in your fat cells to keep them out of your blood and brain. When you start losing weight and the first few pounds come off, the chemicals released from the melting fat cells can cause physical and mental side effects as they circulate in the bloodstream. It's a real turnoff when you are losing weight in order to feel better, but the initial result is that you actually feel worse.

Stress Release

We've all heard the saying "One man's food is another man's poison." It's the same for stress: "One woman's stress is another woman's adventure/learning experience/opportunity for growth . . ." Stress is what you make of it. That's easy to say, until something horrible happens, but you can prepare for stress in lots of ways—prayer, meditation, walking in nature, gardening, hugging trees. These are the "salt of the earth" types of things that people of all ages turn to when things get tough.

There's something to be said, however, for de-stressing all the time. Why wait until things get tough? If you practice de-stressing every day, you will be amazed at how much easier the tough times become. Here are some de-stressing tips that work.

THE DO'S

- Develop an affirmation or mantra—for example: "Every day in every way I am getting better and better."
- Look at your glass as half full and not half empty.
- Rejoice in the beauty and the power of life; take time to "stop and smell the roses."
- Be truthful in relationships, both personal and business.
- Contemplate, pray, meditate, or simply take a walk every day.
- Take time out to play and to laugh.
- Unleash your creativity: Draw, paint, sing, write.
- Listen to relaxing music.
- Exercise: yoga, tai chi, T-Tapp, swimming, walking.
- Get a regular massage.
- Take a relaxing bath with magnesium-loaded Epsom salts (1 cup per bath).

THE DON'TS

- Don't watch TV or violent movies, and you might even cut back on newspapers when you are really stressed.
- Limit your coffee intake.
- Cut out alcohol.
- Cut back on sugar.

Meditation and Stress Reduction

Even a few deep breaths can be enough to reset your body's stress index and turn on your calming chemicals. Often I find myself tense for no reason. I'm cooking or washing the dishes and my abdomen is tight. I take a few deep breaths and release the tension and feel much calmer. Tension is such a learned behavior, but we can easily teach ourselves techniques to overcome the stress. Meditation can be as simple as sitting for five or ten minutes in a relaxing setting. Counting your blessings is something I learned from attending Native American moon ceremonies with a group of friends in New York. In our prayers we gave thanks for everything and everyone on earth.

The Power of Laughter

Look for opportunities to inject humor into your day. I download all the one-liners and jokes I find on the Internet and keep them in a special file called "Open in an Emergency." When I need a lift I just go to my file and start chuckling as soon as I see the title.

One line that I have added to my file came to me when I was writing the section above about how your bloodstream can only handle about one teaspoon of sugar at any one time, while there are ten teaspoons in just one can of soda pop. I began thinking, as I often do, about how people can and do abuse their bodies so badly. Then I just blurted out, "Is the person in charge of my mouth insane?" Other people may not find it funny, but I find it hilarious. It adds a bit of humor to a topic that can become pretty frustrating for someone like me who for the past twenty-five years has been trying to warn people that what they eat does have an effect on their health.

Laughter Is Therapeutic

"Find your own funny bone and stimulate it regularly" is the advice of researchers at Loma Linda University. They have found that laughter reduces stress hormones. It also stimulates the immune system. We now know that stress depletes the immune system, and that the antidote is laughter. Laughter can raise levels of infection-fighting T-cells, disease-fighting proteins called gamma-interferon, and B-cells, which produce disease-destroying antibodies. Laughter also lowers blood pressure and increases muscle strength.

✱ Stress Nutrients

Although we will be tackling diet and nutrients more thoroughly in Chapters 11 and 12, let's look at some specific ways of tackling stress with supplements. The most important nutrients for depleted adrenal glands are vitamin C, the B vitamin pantothenic acid, magnesium, and omega-3 fatty acids. I also used to recommend desiccated adrenal gland supplements from organic animals, but there is some difficulty obtaining such products in the United States.

VITAMIN C

The adrenal glands contain very high amounts of vitamin C, so when they get depleted, vitamin C is depleted as well. Increasing your vitamin C intake by eating several pieces of fruit a day or by taking a natural supplement will help build up the adrenals. Food-based sources of vitamin C are the best. It's also important to use vitamin C products that contain bioflavins—these are equated with the pulp and rind of citrus fruits, whereas ascorbic acid is equated with the juice.

PANTOTHENIC ACID

Pantothenic acid, along with the whole vitamin B complex, is calming for the nervous system but especially the adrenals. However, along with my B complex in my multiple vitamin-mineral, I take pantothenic acid in high doses, 1,000 milligrams once or twice a day, to deal with the stress of a busy life.

MAGNESIUM

Magnesium is my favorite mineral. I wrote a book called *The Miracle of Magnesium* and was amazed at the properties of this simple mineral. It is required for over 350 different enzyme systems in the body, with many of them related to combating stress. Prolonged psychological stress raises adrenaline, the stress hormone, and results in a myriad of metabolic activities, all of which require and therefore deplete magnesium. Magnesium depletion itself stresses the body, which can result in panic attacks, which results in more bursts of adrenaline and creates irritability and nervousness. Not only do our overworked adrenals cause magnesium depletion, but even more adrenaline is released under stress when magnesium levels are low in the body. It's the proverbial catch-22.

When cortisol levels are elevated due to chronic stress, there is less mood-enhancing serotonin produced. And if magnesium is depleted, even less serotonin makes its way to the brain cells, because this mineral is a necessary building block for the production and uptake of serotonin by brain cells. In my opinion, the first line of treatment for someone who is suffering from anxiety or depression is boosting nutrient levels so that the adrenal gland can make enough adrenaline and cortisol, and so the brain can make enough serotonin.

Omega-3 Fatty Acids

Omega-3 fatty acids from flax oil and fish oil are indispensable to the functioning of every cell in the body. Among other things, they form part of the fatty layer of cell membranes. Nerve cells depend on a healthy cell membrane for proper communication of the brain's many neurotransmitters, including serotonin.

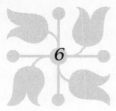

6

Chemicals Called Mom:
The Xenoestrogen Trap

YES, VIRGINIA, CHEMICALS masquerading as hormones can and do stimulate sexual development! Xenoestrogens are mostly chemical substances, such as DDT and DDC, that look just like estrogen. Even plastics look like estrogen, and these chemicals can be stored in sensitive tissues. We know they gravitate to fat cells. These fat cells can be in the breast, for example, where they cause inflammation. Fat cells have a very long life, which means they can stay in your body through your entire life and they can trigger cancer.

✳ Chemicals in the Environment

According to the Environmental Protection Agency (EPA), more than 4 billion pounds of chemicals were released in the United States in 2000. Four hundred licensed pesticides make up 2.5 billion pounds of that total. These chemicals don't remain stationary; with every rainfall they contaminate ground water and seep into wells, reservoirs, and water tables. Another quarter of a billion pounds were "legally" dumped into rivers and lakes by industry that year. Add to that the two billion pounds of air emissions yearly pumped into the air we breathe. In the food we eat, there are thousands of pounds of food additives, and another few thousand pounds of herbicides, pesticides, and food-processing chemicals are found in our diet. Per person, per year, we eat about fourteen pounds of food additives and close to 150 pounds of sugar. Many of these additives are endocrine disruptors, also known as hormone disruptors, and some specifically target estrogen receptors. These are called *xenoestrogens*. Whatever the label, they are bombarding our bodies in a way that has never happened in humankind before.

Who's in Charge of the Environment?

Environment, according to science and medicine, is something that we should control, rather than letting it control us. Unfortunately, science and medicine are sadly mistaken. Here are just a few examples of the results of this type of thinking: industrial effluent polluting rivers and oceans and making fish unsafe to eat; industrial smokestacks polluting the air and giving us acid rain and acid soil; the more than 50,000 chemicals in daily use; food additives; thousands of prescription and over-the-counter drugs; artificial sweeteners; aluminum cooking utensils; household chemicals; pesticides and herbicides; and mercury put in our dental fillings, vaccines, and medicines in spite of knowledge of its toxicity. Let's face it: We are a toxic nation.

We're Loaded with Chemicals

As reported in *Vitality Magazine*, November, 2002, by noted Canadian activist and medical journalist Helke Ferrie: "Our bodies have become the world's toxic dump sites. The billions of dollars' worth of pesticides, plastics, petroleum products, and heavy metal containing technology have made the industrial world rich beyond belief, and threaten human survival as it conquers the earth. As in the story of King Midas, whose touch turned everything to gold— even his wife and children—our economy is killing us." Dr. Sherry Rogers, in her recent book *Detoxify or Die*, pulls no punches. She says, "We have conquered the world with pollution. There are no more pristine areas left without a trace of man's manufacturing might."

Dr. Samuel Epstein, Professor of Environmental and Occupational Medicine, University of Illinois School of Public Health, led the fight to remove DDT from America, although it's still used in other countries. Dr. Epstein maintains in "New Perspectives in the War on Cancer" (Helke Ferrie, *Vitality Magazine*, September 1999) that each one of us harbors 500 different chemicals in all the cells of our body. The Environmental Protection Agency confirms that 100 percent of the world's population harbors traces of heavy metals such as mercury, lead, and cadmium in their blood. Dr. Rogers echoes this warning and writes, "Indeed every living thing now has DDT in its tissues and its toxic effects are increasing over time." Helke Ferrie reports that the World Health Organization admits that, in terms of scientific research on environment pollution, there are no more "control groups" free of toxic synthetic chemicals to be found in the world.

Brain, bowel, and hormonal organs, including testicles and ovaries, are all equally affected. Our bodies ineffectually lash out against the invasion of chemicals that we were never equipped to handle. The result is epidemics of allergies, arthritis, autoimmune disease, cancer, chronic fatigue syndrome, mood disorders, and neurological diseases that, as Ferrie says, "no amount of fancy genetics will explain away" (Helke Ferrie, "Detox or Die," *Vitality Magazine*, Toronto, Canada. October, 2002).

✿ Environmental Medicine

Environmental illness is barely recognized by the medical community; however, the trend of the past decade is to put illnesses caused by environmental factors into the category of "autoimmune disease." In an overly toxic world we are faced with this new designation of illness. This is a non-diagnosis. It has become a catch-all for people who have galloping inflammation in nerves, skin, joints, lymphatic system, endocrine organs, and GI tract. We designate this inflammation as MS, scleroderma, lupus, rheumatoid arthritis, thyroiditis, leukemia, Crohn's disease, and even cancer.

As mentioned in Chapter 3, Dr. Russell Blaylock made it very clear that our definition of autoimmune is not the body attacking a normal self. It wouldn't attack a normal self—it's attacking an abnormal self. It's the abnormality that's at fault, not the body and not the body's immune system. And that abnormality is the buildup of toxins and poisons. The body is attacking the toxins and poisons within us in a desperate attempt to get rid of them, and we must aid that process by regularly and consciously cleansing the body, and not detract from it by giving more medications. Our job with autoimmune disease is not only to treat the disease but, even more importantly, to prevent the toxins from building up in the first place.

When Is Something Toxic?

As mentioned in the Introduction, hormones are measured in nanograms and picograms. So, too, are certain very toxic chemicals. Therefore, a microgram, which is one millionth (1/1,000,000) of a gram, or a nanogram, which is one billionth (1/1,000,000,000), and a picogram, which is one trillionth (1/1,000,000,000,000), can be toxic. Sorry to throw all those zeros at you, but it sure helps to see how powerful chemicals can be at such minuscule doses. It helped me to understand how nanogram measurements of feminizing chemicals in the environment could seriously disrupt the human body. Dr. Theo Colborn, in her book *Our Stolen Future*, described it this way: Think of one part per trillion as equaling one drop of gin in 660 train tank cars of tonic water!

Knowing these numbers also helps to refute the argument from the chemical industry that the amount of chemicals in the environment is too small to do any harm, when in fact it is harmful. To be told that something is not toxic because it is only a "tiny" amount is an excuse that is full of holes.

You don't have to go far to find feminizing chemicals. Many of them are excreted in the urine and feces of the ten million women presently using synthetic estrogens and the tens of millions using synthetic BCP. Estrogens are found in most bodies of water that are tested for the hormone. Industrial solvents, lead, plastics (even the plastic in baby diapers may be a risk), and pesticides are all potential xenoestrogens.

✂ It Began with DDT

Pollution did not begin with DDT, but the first battle to control toxic chemicals began with this well-known pesticide. I heard about the hormonal effects of chemicals when I first became interested in nutrition as a teenager. There was a raging debate about DDT and its adverse side effects. DDT was hailed as a miracle pesticide for protecting U.S. troops in the Pacific by eradicating insects carrying malaria. But, as with most things in our society, we overdid it. We began to use DDT on all our commercial farm products: for vegetables, fruits, and animals; for commercial and home pest-control; and even for mothproofing. Before long, DDT residues were found in cow's milk and human milk, and eventually every person tested had DDT in their body.

Some researchers point out that since the 1940s—the time when estrogenic pesticides such as DDT were first used—the incidence of breast and prostate cancer has doubled and testicular cancer has tripled. Pesticides are also linked to a decline in human sperm counts. Because of the chemical composition of DDT and most other pesticides, they are able to mimic and block the action of estrogen.

Rachel Carson's Legacy

One of the few people who stood up to the onslaught of DDT and toxic chemicals in the environment was Rachel Carson. She wrote her book *Silent Spring* in 1962 and became a shining light of truth for people who were aware of the dangers of pesticides, especially DDT. Through her work and that of other aware scientists such as Dr. Samuel Epstein, DDT was finally banned in America in 1972.

Rachel Carson stated, "For the population as a whole, we must be more concerned with the delayed effects of absorbing small amounts of the pesticides that invisibly contaminate our world." This is still true today—even more so than in the past.

PCBs—Another Threat

In college, I was in honors biology before I decided to go into medicine. In biology we learned that PCBs (polychlorinated biphenyls) were being banned because they were found to be just as dangerous endocrine-disruptors as the recently banned DDT. PCBs were developed by Monsanto and were widely used from 1929 to 1976. Feminizing and masculinizing effects began showing up in animals before they were recognized in humans. A war of studies began, with some showing harmful effects and others, mostly produced by the chemical industry, showing that they were perfectly safe. The public was at a loss to know what to do about these chemicals.

✖ The Wingspread Statement

In 1991, an international community of about twenty scientists published a consensus document that was called the Wingspread Statement. The authors said that they were convinced that the endocrine systems of animals and humans were being disrupted by the bioaccumulation of man-made chemicals. Those compounds—including fungicides, herbicides, and insecticides, industrial chemicals such as DDT and its breakdown product DDE, chlorine, plastics, other synthetic products, and some metals—have the same structure as hormones!

Many of these scientists who worked on the Wingspread Statement had been alerted to these effects during their own study of wildlife populations. However, they also backed up all their observations with laboratory studies that corroborate the abnormal sexual development observed in the field and provided biological mechanisms to explain the observations in wildlife. In their report they gave a long list of evidence supporting their denouncement of endocrine-disrupting chemicals. They found:

- Thyroid dysfunction in birds and fish
- Decreased fertility in birds, fish, shellfish, and mammals
- Decreased hatching success in birds, fish, and turtles
- Gross birth deformities in birds, fish, and turtles
- Metabolic abnormalities (impaired or abnormal use of energy, manufacture of tissue, or handling of resulting wastes) in birds, fish, and mammals
- Behavioral abnormalities in birds; demasculinization and feminization in male fish, birds, and mammals
- Defeminization and masculinization of female fish and birds
- Compromised (impaired) immune systems in birds and mammals

The scientists were able to determine the following four general patterns of effects even though the specific effects would vary among species:

1. The chemicals of concern may have entirely different effects on the embryo, fetus, or perinatal organism than they do on the adult.
2. The effects are most often manifested in offspring, not in the exposed parent.
3. The timing of exposure in the developing organism is crucial in determining its character and future potential.
4. Although critical exposure occurs during embryonic development, obvious manifestations may not occur until maturity.

Regarding the impact of endocrine-disrupting chemicals on humans, the Wingspread researchers reported that the effects of DES (diethylstilbestrol), a synthetic estrogen, are identical to those found in contaminated wildlife and laboratory animals. It is well known that both sons and daughters exposed in utero to DES experience congenital anomalies of their reproductive system and reduced fertility. Putting together all their research and data, the scientists concluded that "humans may be at risk to those same environmental hazards as wildlife."

Scientists Speak Out

Through the Wingspread Statement, and then in a 1995 report in *Scientific American*, the alarm was sounded to the scientific community. Devra Lee Davis, program director for the World Resources Institute, and Leon Bradlow, director of the Laboratory of Biochemical Endocrinology at the Strang-Cornell Cancer Research Center, reported the connection between xenoestrogens and breast cancer.[18] The researchers were puzzled as to why so many women developing breast cancer did not have the usual risk factors such as early onset of menstruation, late menopause, and no children. These three factors increase the total lifetime exposure to estrogen. Excess estrogen is the most common direct cause of breast cancer. It wasn't long before they zeroed in on prolonged exposure to xenoestrogens as the answer to their puzzle.

Bradlow's past research had shown that estrogen can have "good" or "bad" effects in the body. The "good" estrogen (2hydroxyesterone) has no effect on cancer cells. But "bad" estrogen (16alpha hydroxyesterone) seems to trigger normal breast cells to turn cancerous. When Bradlow found that xenoestrogens shift the balance of estrogens in the body toward the "bad" type, he knew this was part of the answer to the cause of breast cancer. Then it just became a matter of testing various compounds for this action. DDT, DDE (a byproduct of DDT), and other pesticides increased the amount of "bad" estrogen in cultured breast cancer cells. However, natural plant estrogens found in broccoli, Brussels sprouts, cabbage, and cauliflower produced the opposite effect.

Davis and Bradlow also theorize that xenoestrogens may bind to estrogen receptors in the cells of the breast, inducing cell proliferation. Some xenoestrogens may also help cells to generate the new blood vessels that tumors need to grow and spread. Another group seems to damage DNA. All of those factors may be at work with the toxic chemical DDT. Dr. Mary Wolff, a researcher at Mount Sinai Medical Center in New York City, measured higher levels of DDT in breast tissue samples of women with breast cancer compared to women without breast cancer.

✎ Our Stolen Future

Our Stolen Future, a book published in 1996 by three concerned authors, Theo Colburn, Dianne Dumanoski, and John Peterson

Myers, brought the truth about endocrine-disrupting hormones directly to the public. The authors' Web site at *www.ourstolenfuture.org* keeps the topic alive with the latest research confirming the chemical-health connection. By reading their book and studying their Web site, you will learn that "endocrine disrupting chemicals alter development of the fetus in the womb by interfering with the natural hormonal signals directing fetal growth. Their impacts, sometimes not detectable until years or decades after exposure, include reduced disease resistance, diminished fertility, and compromised intelligence and behavior."

Some of the recent studies mentioned on their site that caught my eye were the following (included here along with my comments):

Combining xenoestrogens at levels below individual no-observed-effect concentrations dramatically enhances steroid hormone action.

When certain xenoestrogens are measured individually and there seems to be no adverse effects, they are said to have "no-observed-effect." This doesn't mean they are safe, but the chemical industry sometimes implies they are safe if they have no-observed-effect. However, we are not exposed to just one chemical at a time. We are exposed to hundreds, if not thousands, of chemicals, yet for decades they have been studied individually. A series of studies done by Rajapakse and colleagues[19] shows that, when measured together, xenoestrogens have an additive effect that enhances their negative impact on the body.

A yeast estrogen screen for examining the relative exposures of cells to natural estrogens and xenoestrogens.

This paper proves that "the bioavailability of xenoestrogens in serum is apparently greater than that of estradiol," which means that xenoestrogens can have a greater impact (negative) on the body than naturally produced estrogens.[20]

Environmentally relevant xenoestrogen tissue concentrations corre-lated to biological responses in mice.[21]

DDT may have been banned from North America, but it is still used in other parts of the world and we are exposed to it from imported food and from general world contamination. The estrogen-disrupting effects of DDT and HCH (hexachlorocyclohexane) in laboratory experiments with mice were shown to be statistically significant even at levels found in the environment. In other words, they were the levels to which we are all exposed, and not occupational levels of farm workers or chemical workers.

Role of environmental estrogens in the deterioration of male factor fertility.[22]

In this study, infertile men had higher levels of contaminants. It was called a preliminary study requiring more research because of small sample size, but it emphasizes the association between environmental estrogens and male infertility.

✂ Pesticide Research

An international study spearheaded by The Ontario College of Family Physicians found "no evidence that certain pesticides are safer than others—rather, pesticides misconstrued as 'safe' may simply have delayed effects on health." They found links between pesticide exposure and birth defects, fetal death, and many cancers among 12,000 studies reported between 1990 and 2003. They also found that women are more vulnerable than men, because we have a higher percentage of body fat, which is where toxins are trapped.

Children are the worst hit, however, because the toxins affect them during their development. A Greenpeace study titled "Arrested Development" reported in April 2004 that "exposure to even small doses of pesticides impairs children's analytical abilities, motor skills and memory." Lead investigator Kavitha Kuru-ganti said she was shocked by their findings where 898 children exposed to pesticides in agricultural communities were unable to perform simple play-based exercises, like catching a ball or assembling a jigsaw puzzle.

CDC Pesticide Research

The Pesticide Action Network (PANNA), using data from the Centers for Disease Control (CDC), shows that 100 percent of the blood and urine samples that were collected from 9,000 random people showed residues of pesticides.[23] Monica Moore, co-director of PANNA, stated, "This really needs to be a wake-up call. We need to adopt sustainable agriculture techniques. Even if you only eat organic produce, these chemicals are in the air, the water, the stuff you touch. That's why we're calling for removal of these pesticides from the environment."

The Human Experiment

Many years ago I wrote an as-yet-unpublished book called *We Are the Experiment* about my experiences with patients who had chemical sensitivities. These were people who had been to many doctors with a host of symptoms that could not be identified as a specific disease. Prescription drugs made them feel worse, and they were constantly being told that "it's all in your head." Fortunately, I knew something about environmental illness and was able to refer them to the clinical ecologist Dr. Jozef Krop, Fellow of the American Academy of Environmental Medicine. In his recent book, *Healing the Planet*, he lists the following environmental sensitivity and allergy symptoms that his adult patients express:

- *Central nervous system:* fatigue, tension, confusion, hallucinations, hyperactivity, sleep disorders, headache, memory loss, depression, dizziness, numbness, tremors
- *Gastrointestinal system:* heartburn, nausea, bloating, constipation
- *Hematological system:* high or low platelets, anemia, bruising, leucopenia
- *Genitourinary system:* frequency, inability to void, urgency to urinate, prostate problems, infertility, infection of urinary tract, interstitial cystitis
- *Musculoskeletal system:* joint pain, backaches, swollen limbs, muscle weakness, muscle pain, muscle spasms, muscle twitching
- *Respiratory system:* frequent colds, bronchitis, shortness of breath, asthma, heavy chest, sighing respiration
- *ENT system:* nasal stuffiness, sinus infections, watery eyes, earaches, ear infections
- *Skin:* flushing, eczema, cold extremities, rashes, hives
- *Cardiovascular system:* rapid heartbeat, skipped beats, irregular heartbeat, hypertension/hypotension

Endocrine-Disrupting Chemicals

Scientists have learned about the characteristics of endocrine-disrupting chemicals over the past few decades. The following list provides an overview of the major attributes of these chemicals.

1. They persist in the environment—for example, the chemical chlordane has a half-life of forty years, which means that in forty years half of the original amount still exists.
2. Their biological, chemical, anatomical, physiological, and behavioral effects have been observed, researched, and proven on a variety of animal and bird species, and on humans.

3. These chemicals accumulate in animal and human fat cells. They cross the placenta, which results in the fetus actually storing more than the mother. They are also found in breast milk. By 1999, there were a measurable 250 different chemicals in the bodies of people living anywhere in the world.

4. These endocrine-disrupting chemicals are distributed all over the world, by water, air, and food and through migrating birds and fish.

5. Humans are the most affected, because we are at the top of the food chain. The effects are not just additive; through the process of bioaccumulation they increase exponentially as they move up the food chain.

6. Their action on the fetus during crucial stages of development can be toxic at extremely tiny amounts—a fraction of one part per trillion.

7. Endocrine-disrupting chemicals do not act separately; they act synergistically. A weak chemical can be boosted by another weak chemical. The sum of the two is much more than simple addition.

8. Smaller doses actually are more toxic than larger doses. That may be because they act on hormone receptors that can be triggered by one part per trillion.

9. The toxicity of these chemicals can affect the second and third generation in different ways than it affected the first generation.

✴ Xenoestrogen Effects on Sex Hormones

Estrogen in the environment is easier to study in men than women. After all, it just takes a *Playboy* magazine to get a sperm sample from a man, whereas it's a major "operation" to get an egg sample from deep within a woman's ovary! That's why the results of endocrine-disrupting chemicals seem to be affecting more men than women. But don't kid yourself—they are affecting women just as much as men, and are affecting children most of all.

I recently heard the pediatric allergist Dr. Doris Rapp tell a small group of parents of children with autism about the declining sperm count in North America. She pulled no punches in her talk and neither does she in her 2003 book *Our Toxic World: A Wake Up Call*. This hefty volume is "all about chemicals and how they are hurting our children, all wildlife, our planet and us. We have polluted our air, water, soil, food, homes, schools, and workplaces."

Dr. Rapp says that even the cosmetics and personal care products we use every day and put on our skin have ingredients linked to potential health hazards, ranging from chronic fatigue, asthma, and skin problems to a variety of cancers. Dr. Rapp notes how chemicals damage

- Our reproductive system: causing major sexual difficulties and changes in sperm count and fertility
- Our endocrine system: causing thyroid disease, adrenal disease, and diabetes
- Our immune system: causing infections, allergies, and cancer
- Our nervous system: causing learning and behavior problems

You can see that the first two items in this list have a direct impact on hormone balance and must be addressed in any discussion of PMS, perimenopause, and menopause. Knowing these facts means that the symptoms we thought were just "our hormones going awry" actually have a measurable cause. In men, the quality and quantity of sperm has been declining for decades. In women, we seem to have an epidemic of female diseases, much of which can be traced to estrogen dominance and progesterone deficiency.

But don't forget the causes of estrogen dominance discussed in Chapter 4. It's more than just xenoestrogens and endocrine disruptors. It's a combination of:

• ERT, HRT, and BCP in women, and their metabolic products flushed into our water supply
• Xenoestrogens from 100,000 chemicals in our environment
• A poorly functioning liver
• A diet low in natural fiber
• Excess alcohol
• Birth control pills containing estrogen
• Obesity

Pushing Puberty

In Chapter 1, I introduced the topic of premature puberty due to increased estrogen from being overweight and briefly mentioned xenoestrogens. I identified the endocrine-disrupting chemicals that would most affect children as the following: pesticides, herbicides, and insecticides found on their fresh, frozen, or canned fruits, vegetables, and fruit juices; growth hormones in their hot dogs and hamburgers; bovine growth hormone in milk, ice cream, and cheese; estrogen-like compounds used by dentists on children; and even the plastic wrap used on their sandwiches for school lunches.

An article in *emagazine* (November 21, 1997) called "Premature Puberty: Is Early Sexual Development the Price of Pollution?" includes interviews with a ten-year-old and her mother. The preteen is five foot nine inches, and wears a ladies size ten shoe. She's a fully developed woman but still only a child. Her mother blames her daughter's early puberty on her exposure, from the time of conception, to growth hormones and pesticide residues in meat and other foods. And it's not just girls who are affected; the same woman's son was born with only one testicle.

Charlotte Brody, organizing director of the Virginia-based Citizen's Clearinghouse on Hazardous Wastes, is not surprised by the findings. She says, "We've seen this problem before the study came out." She adds, "It's another warning that we are messing with the fundamentals of life, and the weight of evidence points to endocrine disruptors."

Dwindling Sperm

One of the largest studies on sperm counts was conducted in Scotland and presented to the Association of Clinical Embryologists and British Fertility Society in January, 2004.[24] Doing their duty for science, 7,500 men gave a total of 16,000 samples. The results confirmed fears about declining levels of male fertility. The average sperm count of men in Scotland has plunged almost 30 percent in only twelve years. Previous research has shown that over the past fifty years sperm counts around the world have fallen a dramatic 50 percent. Researchers speculate that there could be total male sterility by 2050. While this study didn't evaluate the cause of sterility, previous papers on animals and humans have shown that estrogen can impair sperm. There's incredible irony in the fact that girls are reaching puberty far too early and boys are not reaching puberty at all, in the sense that their sperm don't work.

Menopause and Endocrine Disruptors

Yes, it seems as if another plot is afoot in perimenopause and menopause. It's not "all about xenoestrogens" in menopause.

Endocrine disruptors are disturbing more than just the sex hormones; for this reason, at the time of menopause you could be looking at blocked thyroid function, exhausted adrenal glands, as well as estrogen dominance due to a buildup of xenoestrogens. You can certainly see by now that menopause is not just "a deficiency of estrogen." It's a simple life stage that has become increasingly complex in our toxic world.

Saving the Environment

In answer to the increasing demands by the public to do something about pesticides in our environment, the United Nations has created the Stockholm Convention on Persistent Organic Pollutants (POPs). This is a "global treaty to protect human health and the environment from persistent organic pollutants (POPs)." By definition, POPs are chemicals that:

- Remain intact in the environment for long periods
- Become widely distributed geographically
- Accumulate in the fatty tissue of living organisms
- Are toxic to humans and wildlife

The Stockholm Convention ensures that governments worldwide will "take measures to eliminate or reduce the release of POPs into the environment." The first phase of their recommendations took effect May 17, 2004, and began by banning twelve chemicals, nine of which are pesticides. The accord has been ratified by the required fifty UN member countries. Unfortunately, the United States has refused to sign this treaty.

The Precautionary Principle

Another attempt to curb our chemical appetite has the American chemical industry foaming at the mouth. Reporting for the UK *Guardian* on May 12, 2004, Jeremy Rifkin says that the European Union (EU) is determined to require corporations to prove their products are safe before allowing them to be sold in Europe. He says that they are implementing "the precautionary principle." As the name implies, the precautionary principle doesn't wait for all the *i*'s to be dotted or the *t*'s crossed in scientific analysis. If a chemical or a process is seen by a majority of researchers and studies to be detrimental, then it should be curtailed.

The precautionary principle is something for which Rifkin has been lobbying for decades. It's a term well known in activist circles, but Rifkin says it's "the most radical idea for rethinking humanity's relationship to the natural world since the 18th-century European Enlightenment." Rifkin says that the impact of the adoption of the precautionary principle by the EU ". . . is already being felt within the business community and the halls of government, with profound implications for all of us."

Rifkin encourages the EU's attempt "to establish a radical new approach to science and technology based on the principle of global stewardship of the Earth's environment." He cites an EU document, dated November 2002, that highlighted the precautionary principle that would "allow government authorities to respond preemptively, as well as after damage is inflicted, with a lower threshold of scientific certainty than has been the rule of thumb in the past." Their definition of precautionary principle is ensuring that "'[s]cientific certainty' has been tempered by the notion of 'reasonable grounds for concern.'" The precautionary principle gives government the "flexibility to respond to events in real time, so that potential adverse impacts can be forestalled or reduced while the suspected causes of the harm are being evaluated."

Who's Protecting Us Now?

Presently there are no laws that prevent dangerous chemicals from reaching market. Jeremy Rifkin reports that "99 percent of the total chemicals sold in Europe have not passed through any environmental and health testing review process." But the EU hopes to change all that and make the industry register and safety-test more than 30,000 chemicals at a cost of 6 billion pounds sterling.

Too Many Risks

What spearheaded the precautionary principle in the new EU chemical safety laws is a European debate regarding "the great shift from a risk-taking age to a risk-prevention era." Such a debate does not yet exist in America. Rifkin itemizes the many global risks that are man-made, permanent in effect, and infinitely damaging and costly. Acid rain from chemicals; chemical threat to the Earth's ozone layer; the spread of biological viruses, adulteration of our food supply with chemicals and chemical processing; and the overuse of chemical drugs—all of these seem unstoppable. The Europeans call ours a risk society, and they demand policies that reduce the risks that are still within our control.

In the United States, we've actually taken several steps backward. Our air used to be protected by the twenty-five-year-old "Clean Air Act." However, in 2000 many of those laws were overturned, meaning that industrial plants did not need to improve their filtration systems to allow for cleaner air. By not following through on expected upgrades, industry is allowed to continue to pollute. They will be allowed to let even more toxic pollution flow into our air and into our lives.

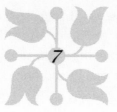

7

Solving the Xenoestrogen Crisis

HERE'S A QUOTE that I love: "The only person who truly welcomes change is a baby with a full diaper." It's from Dr. Richard Earle of the Canadian Institute of Stress. But I have a new way of looking at it. I think that with the overload of information and choices and also the increase in toxicity in our environment and in our bodies, we are all ready to welcome a change!

✿ Women Rule

In my book *Menopause Naturally*, I wrote that statistically women are healthier than men up to the age of menopause. One reason may be that menstrual periods flush toxins from the body along with the accumulation of blood in the uterus. The retention of these toxins, when the period stops, may be a factor in making us susceptible to illness at the same rate as men. Also, as we age, the organs of elimination may not work as efficiently. Therefore, at menopause, women should begin a regular regime of cleansing to take the place of their periods.

Medicine does not focus on proper absorption of nutrients and elimination of body toxicity in dealing with illness. In this chapter, we'll discover why proper digestion and absorption, elimination, and detoxification are crucial to good health and to healing.

✤ Solutions to the Xenoestrogen Crisis

Dr. Theo Colborn, one of the authors of *Our Stolen Future*, says that you start solving the xenoestrogen crisis with your own diet. Being cautious about what you eat is the best way to begin to prevent early sexual development in our children as well as breast cancer in ourselves, because both are related to xenoestrogen exposure. Dr. Colborn recommends organically grown foods and a low-fat diet. She tells *emagazine*, "The ultimate problem here is exposure through chemicals."[25]

We've mentioned several times here that chemicals are stored in fat tissue. Therefore, when you eat animal protein you can ingest chemicals in animal fat. Because the whole food chain is slightly saturated with chemicals, animals that eat contaminated grass, grain, and water or eat other contaminated animals are concentrating chemicals in their bodies. Eating fruits and vegetables sprayed with chemical pesticides, drinking water contaminated with estrogens, and perhaps even breathing air close to chemical factories causes measurable amounts of chemicals in 100 percent of people tested. For these reasons, two items high on the list of recommendations for avoiding chemicals are to cut back on meat and eat organic produce.

But I'm Already Loaded with Toxins

I've been writing and speaking about detoxification for decades. Ever since I realized that the purity of the body was being breached beyond our ability to detoxify, I have advocated safe and gentle ways to cleanse. Cleansing is always the first step in any healing diet or supplement program. Sure, you can start eating organic and take supplements, but if you don't detoxify it's like putting pure water into a dirty pot. The dirt prevails. Let's first clean out the pot.

It's Not Rehab

When most people hear about detoxification they have visions of the Betty Ford Clinic with its drug and alcohol rehab programs. That's why I prefer using the term "cleansing." The body itself has pathways named "phases of detoxification" that are geared to kicking out toxins and poisons. Unfortunately, many of us have overworked our detox pathways to the extent that if we don't help our body out with external detoxification we can get extremely ill. When detoxification is not working as well as it should and foreign chemicals build up, the body stores them away in fatty tissue guarded by immune system cells, which creates area of inflammation.

Addicted to Chemicals

Looking back at Chapter 1, it would be interesting to compare the toxic load of Zorra to that of her friends. Think about women who grow up on antibiotics, the BCP, antihistamines, painkillers, and anti-inflammatories; who predominantly eat processed food, drink sodas with sugar or aspartame artificial sweetener; who use an abundance of strong chemical cleaning products in the home and use lawn chemicals; who buy cosmetics with synthetic additives; and who smoke and drink alcohol. All of these activities cause them to become toxic. When they go to a medical doctor with symptoms of swollen ankles, itchy skin, painful joints, headaches, constipation, and chronic fatigue, their doctor is not going to say, "Oh, Mary, you've just gone and overloaded your body's detoxification systems; we're going to have to put you on a cleanse."

✒ The Body Is Always Cleansing

Medicine pays little heed to the body's detoxification systems. I didn't really learn about them in medical school, nor did I learn about any specific allopathic tests for toxicity. There are no "drugs" to treat toxic overload. Furthermore, drugs, whether prescription or over-the-counter, all must be detoxified in the liver, which places more stress on a system already burdened with an overabundance of chemicals and also stresses the immune system.

The liver functions to detoxify the basic end products of daily metabolism. Most of the biochemical pathways are a little bit like perpetual energy machines, because the enzymes and vitamin and mineral cofactors that are used in the process can be rejuvenated and used all over again. That whole system runs into problems when the body is forced into the extra burden of detoxifying excessive external chemicals. Deficiencies of vitamins and minerals occur, and the detox system can't keep up with the load.

✒ The Liver Works

It is not just a matter of what hormones or how much; the absorption, breakdown, and usage of hormones is of the utmost importance. Hormones are metabolized primarily in the liver. Therefore, a healthy liver is very important if you are on hormone therapy—natural or synthetic. According to New York gynecologist Dr. Richard Walker, estrogens have three pathways in which they can be metabolized—two major: 2-hydroxyestrone (2-H) and 16-hydroxyestrone (16-H), and one minor: 4-hydroxyestrone (4-H). The 2-H system has been shown to produce protective metabolites against cancer formation. Dr. Walker has found that you can enhance the 2-H pathway by eating more cruciferous vegetables (broccoli, cabbage, cauliflower, and Brussels sprouts). Indole-3-Carbinol is a supplement that isolates the most active factor in these vegetables. The 16-H and 4-H pathways have both been found to produces metabolites that are carcinogenic. The 4-H metabolites are the route for metabolizing equine estrogens (Premarin).

The way the liver works to detoxify a fat-soluble pesticide is by converting it into a water-soluble metabolite. The metabolite is usually less toxic, and at least by being water-soluble it can be excreted through the kidneys instead of remaining in the body and stored in fat cells. Toxins stored in fat cells present a special challenge for people who are overweight and go on a cleanse. You have to remember that when fat cells break down during detoxification they liberate toxins that can cause you to feel a bit poisoned. The best advice is to drink plenty of fluids and follow the detox tips given below.

It's also good advice to begin your detoxification slowly and deliberately, and to try to not be overwhelmed by the number of choices. You will begin to feel better when you go on a healthier diet and cut out the chemicals in your life, and you will have more energy to tackle bigger issues. But remember: just take one step at a time. If you are overweight and trying to detoxify, you have to proceed cautiously so that you aren't overwhelmed by all of the toxins being liberated from shrinking fat cells. The feeling of being poisoned causes many people to abandon their goal of losing weight and of detoxifying.

Another word of caution about alcohol. We know that alcoholic men, who have impaired liver function due to alcohol, develop a condition called gynecomastia. This is an estrogen-dominant condition characterized by enlarged breasts, loss of male pubic hair, and eunuch-like features. Women can trigger estrogen dominance not only by drugs and xenoestrogens but also with alcohol. As mentioned earlier, women who consumed two drinks per day had increased blood and urine estrogen levels up to 31.9 percent. Breast cancer risk is higher in women drinkers.

Progesterone's Role in Cleansing

The B vitamins, vitamin C, magnesium, and progesterone are the most important cofactors involved in the process of converting fat-soluble toxins into water-soluble ones. So, if all the information I'm finding about estrogen dominance and progesterone deficiency is true, a lack of progesterone could be one of the underlying reasons why toxins are building up in the body. Estrogen dominance enhances fat accumulation; the overwhelming majority of chemical toxins are fat soluble, so they aim for our fat cells where they are stored. Add to this scenario that a buildup of cortisol due to stress will prevent you from losing weight seems a disheartening conspiracy. However, there are many solutions—and the first one is to detox.

✄ Knowing When Your Liver Is Below Optimum

There are two phases in the way the liver functions. During Phase I, detoxification occurs in liver cell membranes where toxins are subjected to oxidation, reduction, or hydrolysis reactions, which transforms them either into water-soluble products or into substances ready for the Phase II process. The water-soluble substances are eliminated through the urine. Hormones and nutrients help with the transformation and include vitamin B_3, vitamin C, and progesterone. During Phase II, using sulfur amino acids from foods like broccoli and brussels sprouts, along with magnesium, vitamin B_6, B_{12}, and folic acid, those substances that were not rendered water-soluble in Phase I are transformed into a "sticky" substance that can attract other chemicals that help excrete them through the bowels.

If Phase 1 is underactive, even one cup of coffee can rev you up, make your heart race, and keep you awake at night. This means that the liver is falling behind in its detox duties; the resulting buildup of toxicity can lead to impairment of the immune system. If Phase 2 is underfunctioning, when you eat asparagus you get strong-smelling urine and you may be sensitive to sulphites in processed foods.

Enhancing the Phases of the Liver

You can give Phase 1 a helping hand by taking vitamin C, vitamin B, and by getting tested for a progesterone deficiency to see if you need more of this hormone. See page 298 for dosage. To help Phase 2, you need to increase the amount of sulfur in your diet. You know the smell of sulfur from cooking vegetables such as broccoli, cabbage, and Brussels sprouts. Now you know why everyone talks about the healing properties of these "cruciferous" vegetables. It's because they assist the liver in detoxification whether eaten raw or cooked. The other nutrients that assist Phase II detoxification are listed above and include magnesium, vitamin B_6, B_{12}, and folic acid. It is interesting that these four nutrients are also important for the detoxification of homocysteine a recently discovered amino acid that increases the incidence of heart disease. We will talk about homocysteine in Chapters 10 and 12.

Phase 2 detox performs a very important mop-up operation for chemicals that escape Phase 1 detox. Phase 1 detox cannot make petrochemical hydrocarbons, pharmaceutical drugs, and steroid hormones (to name a few) into safer water-soluble chemicals for excretion. These chemicals stay in the body, causing damage until they are bound up by sulfur amino acids (amino acids are the building blocks of protein). Sulfur amino acids grab onto these toxic chemicals and convey a "stickiness" that drags them out of the body. Supplements of sulfur amino acids like methionine, cysteine, and n-acetyl-cysteine (NAC) are being used in detoxification protocols because they are able to pull out toxins such as mercury, lead, and arsenic.

In another phase of liver detox, which is called conjugation, an important body detoxifier called glutathione attaches to the toxic chemical. This metabolic action requires vitamins B_6, B_{12}, folic acid, and magnesium. The most important chemicals neutralized in this process are estrogens, steroid hormones, synthetic hormones, and xenoestrogen chemicals. By now you should have a sense of the importance of detoxification and the need for the right supplements and hormones to do the job. And, remember, the liver also detoxifies excess hormones—even the natural ones.

The Enterohepatic Circulation

The enterohepatic circulation involves bile pigments excreted from the liver that take part in a loop that recycles them back to the liver. Bile picks up the modified toxic chemicals in the liver and travels from the liver down the bile duct into the intestines. If the intestines are healthy, about 90 percent of the bile carrying its toxic load will be excreted in the feces. The remaining 10 percent is reabsorbed back through the intestines and into the liver. If the intestines are not healthy, however, with an imbalance of normal microflora, some of these toxic substances will be reabsorbed and end up in the liver once again, adding to its toxic load.

If some of those bile substances that are reabsorbed back into the liver include natural estrogens, synthetic estrogens, or xenoestrogen, the body is headed for estrogen dominance.

Another impediment to the proper excretion of toxic bile substances is a nasty bacteria that grows in a toxic and constipated bowel. This bacteria produces an enzyme called beta-glucuronidase, which separates estrogen from its neutralizing molecule and points it right back to the liver.

Many toxins—such as petrochemical hydrocarbons, pharmaceutical drugs, and steroid hormones—do not allow molecules to be added or taken away and don't allow themselves to be turned into a water-soluble waste product. Conjugation with glutathione, an important body detoxifier, requires vitamins B_6 and B_{12}, the B folic acid, and magnesium. You can see the delicate orchestration required to cleanse the body: a healthy liver, plenty of vitamins and minerals and progesterone, a healthy bowel with beneficial bacteria, and normal daily bowel movements. If all those factors are not in place, then toxicity—including estrogen dominance—can occur.

Bring on the Solutions

It's only when we agree that toxins are building up in our bodies and are a potential problem that we can turn our attention to trying to get rid of them. If you don't think there's a problem in the first place, how can you find a solution?

The major focus of detoxification is to:

1. Identify the toxins.
2. Decrease your exposure to toxins.
3. Maximize excretion of toxins.
4. Provide nutritional support for specific detoxification pathways.
5. Reestablish intestinal flora balance.

Identify Toxins

We have seen how toxins can permeate our air, food, and water. They are everywhere and in everyone. Measuring them in our bloodstream and urine is becoming more common as testing technology becomes less expensive. In the Resources section I'll mention several labs that do hair, urine, and blood analysis to test for heavy metals and chemicals. (It will be noted which ones require a doctor's lab requisition.) It's probably a good idea to do some measurements before going on a detox program so you know what you are dealing with and so you are able to quantify your progress. Measurements should also include a checklist of symptoms, such as the one used by Dr. Earle that is given in Chapter 5.

⚘ Decrease Your Exposure

Personal cleansing begins with decreasing the toxins you ingest in your daily diet. We'll talk more about diet in Chapter 11, where you'll see how to replace junk foods and empty-calorie foods with a nutrient-dense menu. It's been scientifically proven that by changing to a whole foods diet and getting off the junk, you can dramatically slow down aging and disease. The reason this works is probably because the amount of toxins entering the body is reduced.

Pure Water

Unless you get your water directly from a pure underground water source, you're likely to be drinking chemically treated water from your tap. Enough research exists to show us the dangers of the chlorine and fluoride in our water on a weakened immune system. If you have those concerns, it may be wise to invest in a water purification system. The one you choose should guarantee removal of chemicals, heavy metals, and infectious organisms.

Pure Air

People living in crowded urban environments are exposed to hundreds, if not thousands, of toxic chemicals. However, if you live in a rural farming community, you could be exposed to pesticides and herbicides from crop spraying. And your water supply could be contaminated as well. In a "tight building" that allows little air circulation, you may also be exposed to hundreds of chemicals from your carpets, furniture, paints, varnishes, and cleaning products.

Cleanse Your Home and Garden

While you are focusing on cleansing your body, look at doing the same for your home environment as well. Use chemical-free products wherever possible to reduce contamination. From your bathroom cabinet to your tool shed, do a clean sweep of chemicals. But make sure to dispose of them in an environmentally friendly manner. Most communities have a dangerous chemicals recycling depot that you can contact through the Environmental Protection Agency and the Office of Pollution Protection and Toxics.

✎ Maximize Excretion

You can maximize excretion of toxins by helping the body do its job. We excrete toxins through the bowels, bladder, lungs, and skin. For this reason, the methods of detoxification can include colonics, enemas, herbal laxatives and diuretics, exercise, dry saunas, infrared saunas, steam baths, bathing, sweating, and (for cleaning out the arteries) chelation therapy.

One job of the large intestine is to reabsorb water from the fecal liquid and make it into a solid. Let's follow a heavy meal of greasy fried foods through the digestive tract. Chewing releases enzymes that digest carbohydrates; in fact, about one-third of your carbs can be turned into sugars in your mouth. Next, in the stomach, the main digestive process is the breakdown of proteins by hydrochloric acid. It isn't until the mass of food you just ate arrives near the exit of the stomach and goes into the small intestine that fat enzymes from the pancreas and bile go to work.

Therefore, if you eat a really greasy meal, you'll probably start burping as the fat rises to the top in the churning stomach. Fat slows down the digestion of foods and can lead to incomplete digestion and more burping and intestinal gas. Incompletely digested food is feasted upon by yeasts and bacteria in the intestines, making chemical byproducts with enchanting names such as putrescine and cadaverine—which is described as having the smell of rotting flesh! The longer these chemicals stay in the intestines the more opportunity for them to be reabsorbed into the body as mentioned above.

Colonics in a Clinic

High colonic enemas administered by a nurse or a trained colon therapist are a form of intestinal detoxification. When my grandmother was a nurse in a "fever hospital," high colonic enemas were one of the standard protocols. They were also routinely used before abdominal surgery to ensure a clean bowel. A colonic enema is given while lying comfortably on an examining table. A nozzle is connected to a long tube, which connects to a large container of heated filtered water that is elevated above the examining table. The nozzle is lubricated and inserted into the anus. The water flows through the tube by gravity.

You may be asked to lie on your left side and then on your back as water fills up the large intestine. At any point when slight pressure builds up, the nurse feels this, or you can tell the nurse and a valve is opened allowing the water in your intestines to be released. Over a period of about forty-five minutes the entire large intestine is cleaned. During a detoxification protocol, one or more colonic enemas can be helpful to enhance the process. Make sure you go to a trained colon therapist who uses filtered water and disposable nozzles. An implant of probiotic-beneficial bacteria can be done at the end of a colonic, and you are advised to take oral probiotics to build up good bacteria in your intestines.

Enemas in the Home

Saline enemas, bought in a drugstore, and coffee enemas, prepared at home, are usually self-administered. Coffee enemas are recommended by many doctors—Dr. Nicholas Gonzalas being the most notable—for detoxification while undergoing cancer therapy. Dr. Gonzalas gives himself a coffee enema daily as a preventive health measure. The caffeine, theophylline, and theobromines in coffee are absorbed by the large collection of veins near the anus and cause smooth muscle relaxation in blood vessels and the bile duct. This stimulates the expulsion of bile from the liver and gall bladder, which acts as a flushing laxative through the bowel. It also helps get rid of all the toxins that are attached to the bile without them being reabsorbed.

You can buy a reusable enema bag in a pharmacy. It resembles a hot water bottle with a hose at the end. The recipe for the enema requires filtered water and organic coffee, and following these steps:

1. Boil 4 cups of water.
2. Add 3 tablespoons of coffee.
3. Boil for 3 minutes.
4. Simmer for 20 minutes.
5. Strain and cool to body temperature.

Directions: Make yourself comfortable on blankets covered by a towel on the floor. Learn how to adjust the shut-off valve. Lubricate the nozzle, and then insert into the anus. Lie on your left side and release the valve. Close the valve if you feel pressure, and then lie on your back and open the valve again. Next, move to your right side. Try to retain the coffee for ten to fifteen minutes. A coffee enema is best done after you have had your normal morning bowel movement, and it should not interfere with your bowel movement the next morning.

Exercise for the Lungs, Skin, and Bowels

Anything that makes you sweat is going to help you release toxins. When people do Bikrim yoga that takes place in a 110-degree room, the odor of toxins from people is sometimes overwhelming! When you exercise, deep breathing isn't far behind! It is little known that the lymphatic system, which drains away cellular metabolic wastes, is actively massaged by deep breathing as well as by exercise. Shallow breathing moves air in and out of only a portion of your lungs, but deep breathing can oxygenate twice as much blood by expanding your lungs fully. This fully renewed and revitalized blood brings greater nourishment to every cell in the body.

Exercise also speeds up bowel transit time and encourages detoxification. "Bowel transit time" refers to the time it takes for food to travel from your mouth to your anus. To find out your transit time, have a large portion of beets. Don't be surprised if your urine turns pink, and watch for purple stool. When I was in medical practice, we used to regularly get calls from patients who thought they had blood in their stool. My staff was trained to ask when they last ate beets!

Dry Saunas for the Skin

Although it is called a "dry" sauna, it is important to have some humidity in the sauna, because extreme dryness can irritate the lungs. Saunas make you sweat and sweat carries toxins out of the body. Most health clubs and spas have sauna rooms, or you can install a small sauna in your own home. Here's how it works: Take a shower first and sit on a towel on one of the wooden benches. The upper bench will be hotter, as heat rises. As your skin temperature elevates, your pores open and sweat will trickle down your body. I sometimes rub sea salt over my body, which pulls out even more moisture.

The usual temperature of a sauna is 120 to 150 degrees Fahrenheit. You can create an even higher temperature by throwing water directly on the heating stones to create steam and humidity. Some people claim that a slight elevation of body temperature by one to three degrees mimics a fever that might help protect against viruses and bacteria. It is well known to naturopaths that a fever is one defense against viral and bacterial infection. Beyond helping to detoxify and to prevent infections, the heat itself is relaxing for tired and achy muscles and is beneficial for stress reduction.

After five or ten minutes in the sauna you can cool down with a shower and come back in for another few minutes. This cycle can be repeated several times. You'd be surprised how much sweat you lose in a sauna, so it's very important to drink plenty of water after taking one. Short saunas are beneficial for most people. However, there are special sauna programs using lower temperatures but longer times, under a doctor's supervision, for drug, chemical, and heavy metal detoxification. In New York, more than 100 firemen did sauna therapy as part of a detoxification program funded by Tom Cruise after being sickened in the 9/11 World Trade Center cleanup.

Some precautions: Because heat dilates blood vessels, people with low blood pressure should be very careful to only spend a short time in a sauna and not make the temperature too high. A headache or a feeling of faintness may indicate that your blood pressure is falling. Similarly, if you haven't eaten before your sauna, increased metabolism caused by the heat can drop your blood sugar.

Infrared Saunas

Far-infrared saunas work by directly heating the body, whereas the surrounding air remains relatively cool. Sweating begins quickly and there isn't the discomfort of external intense heat. Infrared saunas are becoming very popular, and I predict that research studies will someday show the benefits of all sauna therapy for detoxification.

Presently, we only have anecdotal reports of people saying they actually smell and feel various chemicals exuding from their pores when they begin sauna therapy.

Steam Baths

Steam baths use wet heat and are the modern version of Native American sweat lodges. The lodges served as ritual cleansing but also cleansed the skin and created a significant amount of sweating, and presumably toxin release, in the process. Steam baths are saturated with moisture and operate at temperatures ranging from 100–120 degrees, whereas sauna baths use dry heat in a range of 175–190 degrees to induce sweating.

Baths

If you don't have access to a sauna or a steam bath, not to worry, as you can still create a spa in your own bathroom. It's preferable if you have a filter on your shower and fill your tub that way to avoid bathing in chlorinated or fluoridated water. Epsom salts acts as a detoxifier in your bath. I use about two cups of Epsom salts myself, but you should start with ¼ to ½ cup. Epsom salts are magnesium sulfate and are absorbed through the skin. Besides being a powerful muscle relaxant, magnesium sulfate is a strong laxative. In my book *The Miracle of Magnesium*, I write about a case of a woman who used so much Epsom salts in a bath that she got loose bowel movements! You can get Epsom salts in most drug stores.

Chelation Therapy

Intravenous chelation therapy is a medical treatment performed in a doctor's office that is thought to improve metabolic function and blood flow through blocked arteries in the body by pulling out heavy metals. I became very excited about the possibilities of chelation therapy when I read a study showing that it could help Alzheimer's patients. As I wrote in *The Everything® Alzheimer's Book*: "We've heard about chelation and its benefits for heart disease, but this was the first report on chelating out amyloid plaque and metals from the brain." A good source for learning more about chelation is the book *The Chelation Way* by Morton Walker.

✄ Provide Nutritional Support

Food, herbs, and supplements can all be used to enhance the body's ability to detoxify. Consider trying the following:

- Eat protein and plants with sulfur amino acids: eggs, broccoli, Brussels sprouts, and cabbage. *Tip:* If you fast during detoxification, you will not have sufficient sulfur molecules to neutralize the toxins that are being released from fat cells and other storage sites.
- Eat vegetables and add fiber to make sure you are having several bowel movements a day to hasten the elimination of toxins.
- Take a multivitamin/mineral supplement, preferably one that is food-based.
- Use mercury detox agents such as chlorella, cilantro, garlic, onions, MSM, N-acetyl-cysteine (NAC), and methionine.
- Use milk thistle herb for liver support during detoxification.
- Use alpha lipoic acid, which is a fat-soluble and water-soluble antioxidant that helps neutralize free radicals and toxins in the body.
- Use glutathione, which is one of the most powerful antioxidants in the body. It is mostly available as an intravenous treatment under a doctor's supervision but is being studied in its sublingual form and in an inhaled form with a nebulizer.

Be sure to discuss all these detox options—including the dosages for your particular needs—with a physician trained in these procedures, such as a naturopath or integrative medicine doctor. Ideally, your cleansing program should be conducted under a doctor's supervision.

✢ Reestablish Intestinal Flora Balance

Probiotics are intestinal bacteria that have a beneficial role in the body. Most people are aware of acidophilus, the common beneficial bacteria found in yogurt. There are dozens of other beneficial bacteria and dozens of research papers showing their benefits to bowel health and general health as well. It's long been thought that probiotics simply worked to protect the gut by a numbers game: the more good bacteria, the less bad bacteria. However, research shows that probiotic bacteria are able to strengthen intestinal immune function and total body immune activity.

✢ A Word of Caution

The major contraindications to detoxification are pregnancy and breastfeeding. You don't want toxins coming out of a long period of storage and getting into your breast milk or going through the placenta. For everyone else there is a general caution. Because there are no routine or inexpensive tests to diagnose toxicity, no one really knows how toxic he or she is, or what the consequences of going on a rigorous detox program might be. When you cut back on meals your body starts breaking down fat cells for energy. When fat is released, so are stored toxins. These toxins then circulate in the blood and make their way into the brain and all other body tissues. Symptoms of brain fog, irritability, anxiety, and even depression can accompany toxins flooding the brain. This is why it's important to seek guidance for your detox program to help you understand the difference between a "healing reaction" and a medical problem.

✁ Cleansing Cancer

In *Hormone Balance*, our discussion of cleansing is focused on battling estrogen dominance and xenoestrogen overload. Estrogen dominance causes a lot of nasty symptoms, up to and including cancer. The following list—"Avoid Known Toxins"—shows you some potentially damaging practices to avoid. The second list—"Do Something Constructive about Toxins"—gives a number of action steps you can take to prevent disease. These two lists are adapted from lists in Helke Ferrie's article "New Perspectives in the War on Cancer."[26]

Avoid Known Toxins

1. Do not smoke, or tolerate smoking in your family's presence.
2. Avoid excessive exposure to sunlight and ultraviolet rays.
3. Do not use breast implants.
4. Do not use dark hair dyes; check out safe alternatives (such as Aveda brand, or henna).
5. Avoid perfumes, perfumed air fresheners, deodorants, and antiperspirants. If they contain benzene, aluminum, or lemon-scented chemicals, or lack a full list of all ingredients to permit a check-up in a toxicology manual, then do not use them.
6. Treat all cosmetic products with extreme suspicion until you have proof positive that they contain no known carcinogens, as safe alternatives exist.
7. Avoid dry-cleaned clothes, and look for nonchemical alternatives.
8. Avoid chlorinated water.

9. Do not drink fluoridated water or use fluoridated toothpaste.

10. Avoid electromagnetic fields, especially with children. Electro-magnetic fields have been linked to childhood leukemia and brain cancers. Use appropriate protection on your computer screen, avoid using a microwave oven, and avoid living near hydro towers.

11. Do not use hormone-disrupting or hormone-mimicking sub-stances such as chemical pesticides, herbicides, fertilizers, fun-gicides, and bug killers such as DEET.

12. Do not use cleaning, polishing, or renovation materials in your home that list unspecified "inert ingredients." If they have toxic warning symbols, require calling a doctor, are "corrosive," give special disposal instructions, or require "well-ventilated areas" for use, then look for substitutes. If you cannot avoid some of these substances (e.g., oil paint, furniture stripper, car mainte-nance materials), wear the best charcoal- filtered mask available and minimize exposure, especially to skin and lungs.

13. Avoid salt-cured, smoked, and nitrate-cured foods.

14. Do not use meat or dairy products from animals routinely treated with antibiotics and raised with hormones. According to Dr. Samuel Epstein, such milk products are among the most effective cancer-causing agents currently known. Safe, certified organic milk and meat products are widely available in health food stores and some grocery stores.

15. Never heat shrink-wrapped foods or put hot food in plastic containers. The plastic molecules migrate into the food when heated. They are xenobiotics—manmade chemicals with struc-tures that are foreign to humans.

16. Avoid food additives, especially Red Dye No. 3, which is found in most junk foods and many soda products. Avoid emulsifiers such as carrageenin.

17. Do not consume hydrogenated vegetable oils, margarine, or trans fats.

18. Limit sport fish consumption to the guidelines provided seasonally by the government.
19. Do not drink or eat foods that contain sugar substitutes such as NutraSweet, aspartame, etc. Avoid refined sugar, as it usually contains silicon. Stevia, unpasteurized honey or maple syrup, and brown rice syrup are healthy substitutes that are easily available.
20. Avoid antibiotics unless your doctor has done the necessary test to identify the exact bacteria this antibiotic kills (except in extreme emergencies, e.g. meningitis); keep any treatment period to a minimum. Learn about natural alternatives.
21. Avoid prescription drugs unless your doctor also gives you a complete list of the drug's side effects; if the drug requires regular liver function tests, insist on discussing alternatives or keep treatment to the minimum.
22. Avoid birth control pills, antihypertensives, antidepressants, and hormone replacement therapy in pill form (toxic to the liver), and do not take tamoxifen preventively. Get the full data on those drugs, and check them out first on the Internet at *www.preventcancer.com*.
23. Do not invest your savings in known cancer source polluters.

Do Something Constructive about Toxins

1. Have your mercury amalgams removed by a dentist trained in the proper protocol.
2. If you are overweight, have your hormone levels checked and find out if you have food allergies, overexposure to estrogen, lack of progesterone, thyroid problems brought on by pesticide exposure, or an adaptation to allergenic foods. Wheat products and refined sugar are also frequent causes of obesity, which promotes cancer through excessive estrogen and pesticide storage.
3. Exercise regularly and moderately.

4. Eat cruciferous vegetables (cauliflower, Brussels sprouts, broccoli, etc.), preferably from organically grown sources; if that doesn't fit your budget, wash all your fruits and vegetables in VegiWash. This will remove pesticide surface residues.

5. Buy your foods in glass containers; avoid cans and plastic.

6. Take supplements, especially vitamins C and E, and minerals such as magnesium. In general, check out the literature mentioned in number 9 and take charge of your health. If you need hormones, consider primarily natural ones and/or transdermally administered varieties in the smallest possible doses—they bypass the liver.

7. Join a health or cancer activist group.

8. Start a pesticide education group in your neighborhood; demand from your local representatives mandatory toxicology disclosure of all chemical ingredients being sold today; approach your local golf course manager and discuss alternative ways of maintenance; go to your city council and get them to explore alternatives to chlorine in public swimming pools and to put a stop to the use of chlorine and fluoride in the water supply.

9. Read the *Journal of Pesticide Reform* for basic information. Some good books to read: Sandra Steingraber's *Living Downstream*, Robert N. Proctor's *Cancer Wars*, Steinman and Epstein's *Safe Shopper's Bible*, and Linda Pim's *Additive Alert*. The 1970s classic by Adelle Davis, *Let's Get Well*, is still an unsurpassed resource. If you have reason to be concerned about cancer, read Dr. Samuel S. Epstein's *The Breast Cancer Prevention Program* (2nd ed.), and give it to your daughters, women friends, and others.

10. If you have been recently diagnosed with cancer, search the Web and the literature for the latest alternative treatments. Your doctor is no doubt sincere, but possibly functions on automatic pilot, especially if he or she relies on drug representatives instead of the medical journals.

11. Only a determined consumer revolt and informed resistance will turn the cancer tide.

The Dirty Dozen

A great summary of what to avoid is the following list that Dr. Samuel Epstein calls "The Dirty Dozen"—thirteen toxins you can choose NOT to use, from his *The Politics of Cancer Revisited.*

1. All contraceptives, hormones, HRT
2. Food additives: aspartame, food dyes, fluorides
3. Premenopausal mammography
4. Heavy metals: mercury, lead, cadmium, arsenic, aluminum, nickel
5. Silicon implants
6. Animal fats from animals that are fed hormones and antibiotics
7. Estrogenic pesticides, which cause estrogen dominance
8. Bovine growth hormones injected into dairy cows and contaminating milk
9. Household chemicals, cosmetics
10. Lindane lice shampoos
11. Workplace carcinogens
12. Lifestyle risks, such as alcohol, tobacco, and dark hair dyes
13. X-rays in pregnancy and childhood

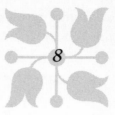

8

Perimenopause: A New Disease?

SEVERAL AUTHORS HAVE WRITTEN that perimenopause is a contrived disease—and I agree. While writing this book, I shared this notion with Susun Weed, the well-known herbalist. She immediately told me a fascinating story about the actual invention of the word "perimenopause."

✳ The Invention of Perimenopause

While on a menopause panel a few years ago, Susun and several of the women panelists were enthusing about the "power of menopause" and extolling women to call their hot flashes "power surges" and not get pulled into the "medical-media hype" of labeling menopause a disease.

An older male gynecologist, also on the panel, felt he was doing women a service by labeling menopause an illness and offering the "cure" of artificial hormone replacement. He became very annoyed because the women there were not taking him seriously. After the panel, he told Susun and a handful of women that he was going to take the wind out of their sails by inventing a new word. Susun didn't quite know what he meant and asked, "What do you mean, invent a new word? How can you do that?" He said he was going to not only invent a new word but also a new disease—one called "perimenopause."

As a result, we women are now defined by our hormones from birth to death. We are living in one of several hormonally related disease categories all through our lives: precocious puberty, puberty, PMS, pregnancy, perimenopause, or menopause.

The Elusive Definition of Perimenopause

As for the definition of perimenopause, I couldn't find one in my medical dictionary. My 1993 edition of *Taber's Cyclopedic Medical Dictionary* had never heard of perimenopause. The most recent edition of *Dorland's Illustrated Medical Dictionary* calls perimenopause "the time just before and after menopause" and also notes that "there are noticeable drops in estrogen levels for three to five years prior to menopause."

Dorland's is using the term "peri" to mean "around the time of," or more simply premenopause, which is the term that most doctors have been using for decades for the time before menopause. However, the statement that there are "noticeable drops of estrogen three to five years before menopause" is probably in error, as shown in our discussion below of the work of Dr. Jerilynn Prior.

Most women slip gradually into menopause, except if they have had surgical removal of their ovaries. Menopause is an event that medicine tells us is defined by the cessation of periods for one year after normal changes in ovarian function. Perimenopause is even less defined. It seems that any menstrual irregularity from the ages of thirty to fifty could fit into the new definition of perimenopause.

By changing the name premenopause to perimenopause, indeed, a new disease condition was invented. Despite its recent arrival in the lexicon of medicine, a May 2004 PubMed search for "perimenopause" that I performed was able to turn up a startling 27,756 citations! In the past decade we have witnessed the marketing strategy of "Create the disease and offer the cure." Reading the North American Menopause Society guidebook from May 2003, I see that the basics of menopause are allotted four pages, whereas perimenopause nets a total of nineteen.

Another View on Perimenopause

Dr. Adrienne Fugh-Berman from the Georgetown University School of Medicine co-wrote an article for Janine O'Leary Cobb's wonderful menopause newsletter *A Friend Indeed*. In the article, titled "Perimenopause: An Invented Disease," she and her co-author called it the "latest media event" and "another time in a woman's life when the characteristics of her menstrual cycle give her a chance to be considered abnormal." In their opinion, "Perimenopause increases both the number of women eligible for unnecessary tests and treatment, and the duration of their eligibility for special attention from pharmaceutical companies."

What Is Perimenopause?

The amount of information and advice on perimenopause could fill volumes. (I'll be adding to that pile by discussing it myself!) Obviously, however, it doesn't matter that it's a made-up word when so many women in the premenopausal years feel out of balance. But instead of defining it by a lack of hormones and using hormone replacement therapy, let's go into the reasons it happens and how we can treat it without necessarily using synthetic HRT.

Whether it is due to too much estrogen or not enough progesterone, or a combination of both, or for other reasons, several authors have listed the following as the most common symptoms of perimenopause:

- Menstrual irregularities
- Menstrual cramps
- Heavy periods
- Light periods
- Hot flashes
- Night sweats
- Vaginal dryness
- Vaginal thinning

Other symptoms that may by related to hormonal fluctuations but are not as common are:

- Acne on the face
- Anxiety
- Bloating
- Breast tenderness
- Changes in processing information
- Decrease in arousal and orgasms
- Decreased libido
- Depression
- Fatigue
- Hair growth on the face
- Hair loss on the head
- Headaches
- Heart palpitations
- Irritability
- Joint pains
- Memory loss
- Migraines
- Mood swings
- Nausea
- Skin changes
- Sleeping problems
- Urinary incontinence
- Urinary tract infections
- Urinating more frequently
- Weight gain

The Hallmark Symptoms of Perimenopause

The most common scenario for perimenopause, which is usually noted in retrospect, is to have flooding periods for several months before skipping a few. This pattern can repeat itself many times over several years. Worsening PMS seems to be the other symptom of perimenopause that gets women's attention. High estrogen levels plus stress hormones and not enough progesterone conspire to make women feel like they have PMS all month.

Estrogen Excess in Perimenopause

Jerilynn Prior, M.D., is a professor of endocrinology and metabolism at the University of British Columbia in Vancouver, B.C. She also heads up a one-of-a-kind research institute called the Centre for Menstrual Cycle and Ovulation Research. Dr. Prior reminds us that out of the many symptoms I've listed above, "Not one of these symptoms is specific to the 'perimenopausal.' Instead, the list is a compilation of symptoms attributed variously to menopause, menstrual cycle changes, pregnancy—and just being a woman." She goes on to decry the fact that having perimenopause as an emerging health condition gives doctors the notion that if you miss one period, are over thirty-five, and have a few of the above symptoms you are entitled to a prescription for HRT. In one of her articles, Dr. Prior calls perimenopause "The Ovary's Frustrating Grand Finale."[27]

Dr. Prior shares her personal experience with a very rough perimenopause, which is what propelled her to fully research the condition. She discovered that, contrary to popular medical opinion, estrogen levels are on average higher than normal during perimenopause. Since medicine views menopause as a deficiency disease, then it only stands to reason that the years leading up to menopause will show a decline in estrogen levels. However, that theory was not born eout in scientific research.

Dr. Prior found evidence for this groundbreaking information by analyzing over a dozen studies that measured hormone levels in perimenopausal women. Although the individual studies tried to make the case that estrogen levels were dropping, when accumulated and averaged the levels were actually significantly higher in perimenopause than in women in their twenties and thirties.

Fluctuating Estrogen

Dr. Adrienne Fugh-Berman of the Georgetown University School of Medicine agrees that estrogen levels in the years leading up to the menopause are more often high than low. She cites the variability of estrogen in those years as the reason for perimenopause symptoms. Women can go through their twenties and thirties with no noticeable hormonal symptoms, and then in their forties start having breast tenderness and mood changes, especially around their periods. It's as if the low estrogen times are lower, with hot flashes at the beginning of the menstrual cycle, and the high estrogen times are higher, causing breast tenderness before the period. These women "have it all."

I remember a patient who developed migraines that occurred before her period and no one could figure out the cause. Because they were premenstrual, we all knew they were hormonal. But twenty years ago, proper hormonal testing was either not available or prohibitively expensive. Her gynecologist put her on Premarin, which made them worse. Today, I realize she was estrogen dominant and needed to lower her estrogen levels and raise her progesterone.

It is indeed a hormonal roller coaster for some. Dr. Fugh-Berman, however, reminds us that young girls do not have hot flashes that go along with their low estrogen, so it's not specifically low estrogen that causes those symptoms but rapid cycles of falling and rising estrogen levels. Dr. Jerilynn Prior tells the story about her first hot flash. She was still menstruating regularly with no sign of hormonal imbalance. Then one morning she woke up very early feeling very angry. She said her heart was pounding and her legs were twitchy and she was in full fight-or-flight mode. That changed abruptly into a wave of heat that left her weak and shaken. The next day her period started. This is a clear example of how hot flashes are related to a rapid drop in estrogen, which is what occurs to trigger the onset of menses.

In my practice, most women in premenopause with mild symptoms of hormonal imbalance were relieved to know that their hormones were just bouncing around and they stopped worrying about them. For some women, whose symptoms were more severe, making adjustments to diet and lifestyle and adding supplements brought balance.

Progesterone Deficiency in Perimenopause

With all this talk about estrogen, we can't forget about progesterone. I remember in my practice women in their mid-thirties talking about a change in their periods. After twenty years of regular cycles that they could set their clocks by, they suddenly began to have longer or shorter cycles and more or less bleeding. There was also a group of women who began to develop fibroids and ovarian cysts. It's only now, as I step back and look at the patterns, that I can understand that some of the symptoms were due to estrogen dominance and some were due to progesterone deficiency, which are actually both sides of the same coin.

As the ovaries age and produce fewer eggs, there are months when there is no one egg that goes on to produce progesterone. These anovulatory cycles lead to diminishing levels of progesterone. With estrogen continuing to be produced by newly stimulated eggs each month, estrogen levels remain elevated. Compared to progesterone, estrogen may actually appear excessive, leading to estrogen dominance. Add to that the xenoestrogenic effect of chemicals that enter the body and you have a true hormonal imbalance.

Remember that progesterone is a calming and relaxing antidote to estrogen, countering many of its effects at the cellular level and in the nervous system as well. The calming effect of progesterone is especially missed when you are also under increased stress, which causes increased elevation in the stress hormones adrenaline and cortisol.

⚕ Diagnosing Perimenopause

In medicine, to have proof that a disease exists and to accurately diagnose it, you need specific tests or measurements. In the case of perimenopause, when doctors try to find evidence of the condition they usually sample the two main hormones that go out-of-range in menopause, estrogen and FSH. Because estrogen swings widely in a normal menstrual cycle (as you can see in Figure 4.2 on page 74), estrogen has high points and low points throughout; for this reason, it doesn't work as a one-time measurement. And, as Dr. Prior found, perimenopausal women have, on average, higher levels of estrogen in the years prior to complete cessation of their periods.

What about FSH?

FSH stands for *follicular-stimulating hormone*, and its job is to stimulate the ovaries to the point of producing an egg every month for a potential pregnancy. When an egg forms in the ovary there is a feedback signal to the pituitary to stop producing FSH. But if an egg does not form, FSH keeps trying to stimulate the ovary and eventually the ovary becomes less sensitive to FSH in general.

The reasons why an egg does not form may include age, or a variety of endocrine-disrupting chemicals creating a cycle of imbalance, which disrupts FSH. When ovulation does not occur, there is an abnormal period—one that is often absent or weak, though if there is too much estrogen compared to progesterone then bleeding could be heavy.

Aging ovaries are not about FSH diminishing, as FSH levels get higher as the ovaries get less sensitive. When estrogen is low (as happens when no eggs are maturing in the ovaries), the production of FSH by the pituitary increases. An increase in FSH stimulates eggs to ripen and mature for ovulation. With menopause, FSH levels continue to rise. FSH keeps pounding harder and harder at the door to the ovaries but can't get in. It's these high levels of FSH that ultimately are used to diagnose menopause. With the new disease condition of perimenopause, doctors are trying to quantify exactly how much FSH you need to have to qualify for this new condition.

The FSH Test—Useless for Perimenopause

According to Dr. Adrienne Fugh-Berman, determining a woman's condition from the FSH test is not that easy. She says, "This is a useless test for this purpose, although perhaps appropriate for an invented disease." In her opinion, "The primary purpose of the blood test is ceremonial: it allows health care providers to make scientific-sounding pronouncements." Dr. Fugh-Berman also agrees with Dr. Prior that estrogen levels are not necessarily low in the years leading up to menopause. And as the estrogen levels fluctuate widely, so do the FSH levels. A one-time test of either estrogen or FSH could show results that could be completely different within a few hours.[28]

What about Ultrasound?

Used in every modern-day pregnancy, and now to determine fertility, it won't be long before ultrasound will become the diagnostic tool of perimenopause. Actually, that was a bit tongue-in-cheek, but it's not far from the truth. The well-known British medical journal *Nature* published a study in June 2004 entitled "Ultrasound Test Predicts 'Reproductive Age.'" If you've ever taken biology you know that a woman is born with a finite number of eggs without the possibility of creating any more. It's not as bad as it sounds, because we are born with several million, but over time, the number of eggs diminishes and the ovaries get smaller.

Because many working would-be moms have put their biological clock on mute, they are asking doctors how much longer they have before their clock stops and they run out of eggs. You can't directly count the number of eggs left in the ovary. However, that question has now been answered with a study that measures ovary size and equates that with the number of remaining eggs. For fertility clinics, this new method of testing can let a woman know her potential chance of getting pregnant without having to resort to fertility drugs that prod the ovary to give up some extra eggs for the cause.

Research has shown that at menopause there are only about 1,000 eggs left huddled in each ovary. Researchers on the ultrasound study have said they would now be able to diagnose menopause by the size of a woman's ovaries. In fertility blood testing, blood hormone tests are not accurate enough to indicate how many eggs are left. It's the same in perimenopause where estrogen levels are not enough. Perhaps several thousand eggs will become the diagnostic cut-off for perimenopause.

✒ The Causes of Perimenopause

There are many different factors at play that can determine the quality of perimenopause, and there is no one single cause for it. The most important factors tend to be diet, stress, and xenoestrogens. When estrogen and progesterone dance to the tune of stress and chemical disruption, they can fluctuate wildly and then gradually decline as we age. Aging brings its own "blessings"—wisdom and memories—but also the possibility of weight gain and declining organ function—thyroid and adrenals, especially. In Chapter 6, you read how xenoestrogens mimic estrogen; in Chapter 5 you saw how stress affects our hormonal balance; and you now have some idea about toxins stored in fat. In perimenopause, unfortunately, all these problems add up.

Don't forget the ongoing stress of relationships at home and at work. Positive or negative stress can have a strong effect on the body. A friend of mine who got married in her forties said her periods completely shut down for four months after her wedding. They did come back again, but she had a taste of perimenopause entirely due to stress. Job stress is another important factor, whether it's good stress or bad. Both deplete the adrenal glands of important stress hormones.

Fat Findings

As mentioned earlier, cholesterol is responsible for making our hormones. Natural estrogen hormones are created using cholesterol stored in our fat cells. Those extra pounds that appear as we get older—the ones that stick to you no matter how much you diet—may, in fact, be the body's way of getting more hormones. It's a survival mechanism that is locked in our genes—and, yes, it often makes our jeans bulge!

Unfortunately, our genes haven't caught up to the fact that we are already 60 percent overweight as a nation (though our jeans have probably figured this out by now). We really don't need help in gaining weight; we need help in losing it. Our genes also don't know about xenoestrogens and other toxins that are taking up residence in fat cells and making us retain fat. We'll talk about diet in Chapter 11 to help you understand the importance of good fats and how to limit bad fats.

Stress Factors

Excessive stress diverts the adrenal glands toward the production of adrenaline and cortisol and away from their function of supporting estrogen production. The higher the cortisol the less estrogen! Wait a minute, you may say, doesn't that seem to contradict what I've been saying about estrogen dominance? But it's not a case of simple addition and subtraction. Natural estrogens can be low in the blood, but if progesterone is also low then estrogen is higher in relation to progesterone and that's what counts. Also, xenoestrogens can mimic estrogen in the body, stimulating estrogen receptor sites and causing estrogen adverse reactions but not beneficial estrogen effects.

When I talked about the adrenal glands in Chapter 3, I mentioned that high cortisol results in excess production of insulin. The end result of too much cortisol, excessive insulin, and frequent bursts of adrenaline is a combination of weight gain, bloating, tender breasts, heavy bleeding, premenstrual migraines, hot flashes, night sweats, anxiety, and insomnia. The additive effects of daily stress can be just too much to handle. With such a combination of factors, just because you are a certain age, perimenopause is said to be the cause, whereas it is more likely a combination of stress, estrogen dominance, progesterone deficiency, excess adrenaline, cortisol, and insulin—and all the various reasons for creating those imbalances in the first place. Whew!

Xenoestrogens

It's unfortunate that there are no readily available and inexpensive tests for diagnosing xenoestrogen load in your body. Knowing whether your hormonal imbalance is due to these chemicals could help focus you on a more specific treatment program. In the meantime, Chapter 7 on treating xenoestrogens and Chapters 11 and 12 on diet and supplements will give you some direction to help eliminate xenoestrogens.

A Word about Candida

Estrogen dominance can cause the overgrowth of the common intestinal yeast called *Candida albicans*. We know that because yeast vaginal infections get worse just before the period when estrogen levels are highest, as seen when you're on the birth control pill or ERT. If you happen to take antibiotics along with estrogen pills, you can stimulate a real yeast overgrowth, because antibiotics kill off the bacteria in the intestines and leave lots of room for yeast to grow both in the intestines and in the vagina. Even a diet high in sugar, white flour products, and dairy can stimulate yeast overgrowth. Alcohol is another trigger to yeast growth.

Candida albicans produces up to 178 different antigenic byproducts that can act as toxins and stimulate allergic reactions in our bodies. One of these is a pseudoestrogen that can either block or mimic estrogen effects. Others are alcohols and aldehydes that can cause such extreme symptoms as drunkenness. If you drink alcohol and have yeast overgrowth, you can feel more drunk or appear more drunk because you are already making your own brew! Even worse, we now know that hormone imbalance can be a direct result of the overproduction of Candida organisms. Research shows that Candida antibodies cross-react with ovary tissue, thyroid tissue, and adrenal tissue. This means that Candida antibodies can attach to these tissues and jam their action, leading to hormone dysregulation. Candida can definitely worsen perimenopausal symptoms.

Candida symptoms can be identified with the following Candida questionnaire adapted from Dr. William Crook's book *The Yeast Connection and Women's Health*. If your answer is "yes" to any question, circle the number that follows the question. When you've completed the questionnaire, add up the points you've circled. Your score will help you determine the possibility (or probability) that your health problems are yeast related.

1. Have you taken repeated or prolonged courses of antibacterial drugs? (4)
2. Have you been bothered by recurrent vaginal or urinary tract infections? (3)
3. Do you feel "sick all over," yet the cause hasn't been found? (2)
4. Are you bothered by hormone disturbances, including PMS, menstrual irregularities, sexual dysfunction, sugar craving, low body temperature, or fatigue? (2)
5. Are you unusually sensitive to tobacco smoke, perfumes, colognes, and other chemical odors? (2)
6. Are you bothered by memory or concentration problems? Do you sometimes feel "spaced out"? (2)
7. Have you taken prolonged courses of prednisone or other steroids; or have you taken "the pill" for more than 3 years? (2)
8. Do some foods disagree with you or trigger your symptoms? (1)
9. Do you suffer from constipation, diarrhea, bloating, or abdominal pain? (1)
10. Does your skin itch, tingle, or burn; or is it unusually dry; or are you bothered by rashes? (1)

Scoring: If you are a woman whose score is 9 or more, your health problems are probably yeast-connected. If your score is 12 or more, your health problems are almost certainly yeast-connected.

Delayed Pregnancy

We look to scientific studies to help formulate our opinion on how to live our lives. However, when it comes to delayed pregnancy, I have not encountered any studies that define what a late pregnancy can do to our hormones. In my experience, women who had their first child later in life have less resilience and more hormonal problems than a younger mother. First of all, the delivery is usually much more difficult in a woman in her late thirties and forties compared to one in her early twenties. The ligaments in the pelvic area are not as loose and pliable. Often a late pregnancy will result in a cesarean section rather than natural childbirth. A surgical procedure adds the stress of recovery from an anesthetic and a wound healing. I have diagnosed hypothyroidism in most late pregnancies, as the thyroid is being called upon to do extra duty. For all these reasons, a delayed pregnancy can result in perimenopausal symptoms that are partly due to depleted adrenals and overworked thyroid.

✣ Saying Goodbye—The Emotions of Perimenopause

Dr. Jerilynn Prior, in her article "The Ovary's Frustrating Grand Finale," shares her own perimenopause story.[29] It all started when she began to have dreams of having a baby when she turned fifty. She said she had two children and absolutely no thought of becoming pregnant. Then she realized her dreams were a way of closing the door on that chapter of her life. Many women, whether or not they have had children, feel the sting of that loss and incorporate those feelings into their overall perimenopausal symptoms. If you are particularly upset about losing your fertility you may experience more physical and emotional symptoms at this time.

Dr. Prior realized that in her dreams she had the same symptoms as she was experiencing in real life. She realized she had estrogen dominance with symptoms of swollen and tender breasts, increased vaginal mucus, and a heavy, crampy feeling in her uterus. She further realized that the problems that women are having in their perimenopause are probably due to estrogen dominance and progesterone deficiency.

Other losses imprinted on women in our society are those of sexuality and beauty. Wrinkles reflect the loss of superficial beauty, maybe, but inner beauty is something that can be cultivated and can grow as we age. Many women talk about perimenopause and menopause as a time for a face-to-face, honest appraisal of their lives.

⚘ Medical Treatment for Perimenopause

Unfortunately, when perimenopause is defined as a medical condition with falling estrogen, the obvious treatment offered is hormone replacement. Because of the negative effects of ERT and HRT in the recent large-scale studies that you read about in Chapter 1, doctors are being advised not to prescribe these therapies except to women having severe menopausal symptoms. However, there is no such prohibition on the use of the birth control pill (BCP) in perimenopause. In fact, that seems to be the medical treatment of choice. By the way, BCPs are simply another form of synthetic hormone replacement. According to Dr. Christiane Northrup, "They are widely used during perimenopause to mask symptoms."

⚘ Seasonale for Perimenopause

Create the disease and offer the cure. The latest "cure" for perimenopause, according to marketers of Seasonale, is a new birth control pill that "lets" women have only four periods a year. As I mentioned earlier, I attended a teleconference for doctors just before Seasonale was launched in November 2003. The focus of this new way of taking the BCP was on younger women, but emphasis was also placed on perimenopause and the use of Seasonale for women right into their menopausal years. As one doctor put it, women can take Seasonale right up until they start HRT. In medical school I was taught that women should only take the BCP for a maximum of ten years and then find other means of contraception. Now, Seasonale is being marketed for women from age thirty-five to fifty-five.

Side Effects of Seasonale

In addition to the side effects of the BCP listed in Chapter 1, which include blood clots, strokes, and heart attacks, "breakthrough" bleeding occurs more in Seasonale. In a report on Seasonale in the *Virginia-Pilot*, Liz Szabo talked about the concerns of many women's groups about the impact of Seasonale on the population. In one study, women bled as much on Seasonale as on the monthly BCP when all the days of breakthrough bleeding were added up. A reported 7.7 percent of women dropped out of Seasonale studies because of "unacceptable bleeding." This was compared to 1.8 percent of women taking monthly BCP. The fact that breakthrough bleeding could not be predicted like an ordinary monthly period was an added aggravation. One of my concerns is that the "unacceptable bleeding" with Seasonale will propel the drug company to make an even stronger pill to keep bleeding from happening at all.

Uterine Stimulation

The lining of the uterus builds up due to the constant stimulation of hormones, and when it is not released, as it would be with a monthly pill, breakthrough bleeding can occur. The body in its wisdom wants to shed this lining. One of the major criticisms of the continuous use of BCP is that the estrogen in the BCP is constantly stimulating the uterine lining. In ERT, constant estrogen stimulation of the lining of the uterus leads to uterine cancer. And the use of a synthetic progesterone pill did nothing to prevent it.

In another ten years are we going to hear that the BCP causes cancer when used for more than ten years? Will Seasonale, used continuously with only four breaks a year, be enough to shed an abnormal uterine lining? Eastern Virginia Medical School, where Seasonale was developed, only followed 682 women taking either Seasonale or regular monthly pills for one year. That means only 341 women took the continuous pill. This is not enough of a sample or a long enough duration to determine long-term effects.

Are Periods a Mistake?

The National Women's Health Network cautions that promoters of Seasonale convey the false impression that having fewer periods is somehow healthier. It says this is the wrong message to impart to young girls. Seasonale marketers imply that a synthetic hormone is the treatment for cramps, irregular bleeding, and other menstrual problems, including PMS. Women may feel they are being chided for putting up with these symptoms rather than suppressing them with a pill.

According to Dr. William E. Gibbons, chairman of the Eastern Virginia Medical School department of obstetrics and gynecology, Seasonale "makes menstruation optional. There isn't any definitive reason why women should have a period at all."

Faulty Research

Liz Szabo found that the Society for Menstrual Research, an interdisciplinary group that studies all aspects of menstruation, demanded more research on the continuous BCP. According to them: "Studies should include women who are not taking any oral contraceptives and not just compare women on different schedules of active pills." A 100-woman survey by Ingrid Johnston-Robledo, a psychologist at the State University of New York at Fredonia, found that women were indeed worried about the continuous use of birth control hormones. They were concerned about short-term and long-term side effects, as well as repercussions on their future fertility. Dr.

Johnston-Robledo expressed apprehension about the negative characterization of regular cycles of menstruation as impairing women's work productivity and heightening emotions such as "depression, distrust, and aggression."

✕ Natural Treatment for Perimenopause Complaints

In Chapters 11 and 12 we'll discuss the diet and supplement approach for both perimenopause and menopause. In this chapter, I'll outline natural treatments for perimenopause-specific complaints. When I talk specifically about menopause, in Chapter 9, I'll focus on some menopause-specific complaints that may also occur in perimenopause.

Flooding Menses

Flooding periods are not only a nuisance but they can also lead to enough blood loss to cause anemia. I learned in medical school that if you soak through at least twelve pads or tampons during one whole period you are losing too much blood, along with too much iron for your normal diet to replace. In that situation, you need to take an iron supplement.

Instead of using iron tablets, which invariably cause constipation, I recommend foods that are high in iron such as liver, green leafy vegetables, and almonds. Also recommended are formulas that combine the mineral iron with vitamin C for enhanced absorption, along with other blood-building nutrients such as the whole B complex, vitamin A, vitamin E, and copper, as well as iron-rich herbs. Herbs that are high in iron include yellow dock, dulse, kelp, dandelion, parsley, and nettle. By diversifying your iron sources, you will just need to look for a formula with 20–30 milligrams of iron instead of the usual 300 milligrams per dose. In my practice I had great success with bioflavinoids such as rutin and hesperitin to help strengthen blood vessel walls so they would clamp down properly at the end of a period and not allow excessive bleeding.

What is most important to know about flooding periods is why they are occurring in the first place. They are usually due to estrogen dominance. Balancing the levels of progesterone and estrogen is the definitive treatment for flooding periods. We'll talk more about progesterone therapy in Chapters 12 and 13.

Fibroids

Another reason for heavy periods is the presence of fibroids in the uterus. These benign growths occur in the walls of the uterus; they are made up of the same cells but form dense tumors that can vary in size from an orange to a melon, or even larger. Fibroids stretch the lining of the uterus and cause more tension on the blood vessels and consequently more bleeding. Again, the main cause of fibroid growth is estrogen dominance. We know from looking at the effects of estrogen on the body (see Figure 4.2 on page 74) that estrogen causes the lining of the uterus to build up. The size of the uterus therefore increases. During anovulatory cycles the uterus enlarges because it doesn't have enough progesterone to cause shedding of the lining.

With estrogen dominance due to anovulatory cycles, a buildup of xenoestrogens, and a toxic liver, the whole uterus can increase in size with or without fibroids and cause pressure on other internal organs. Pressing up against the bladder can cause frequent urination, and pressing against the bowel can cause diarrhea or constipation.

With menopause, fibroids begin to shrink. That sometimes is not an option for many women. Unfortunately, most doctors view fibroids as a surgical condition. They are not aware of the role of estrogen dominance in the creation of fibroids. They also argue that a fibroid is too embedded in the uterus to dissect it free of the uterus.

A small number of gynecologists have proven that argument wrong. Fibroidectomy does take more time to perform than a hysterectomy, and some doctors will not spend the time necessary to do a careful dissection of a fibroid tumor. However, if the problem with bleeding or pain from fibroids is severe, balancing hormones is the first step—one that should be taken long before considering surgery. We'll be talking about hormonal testing and treatment for both perimenopause and menopause in Chapter 13.

SUPPLEMENTS FOR HEAVY PERIODS AND FIBROIDS

Dr. Tori Hudson, professor at the National College of Naturopathic Medicine, Portland, Oregon, is one of the foremost women's health experts in the United States. She says, "Natural therapies are very well suited for the perimenopausal woman. . . . Conventional hormone therapy (HRT or ERT) is not the only option available." As you will read in much more detail in Chapter 12, there are a host of supplements and herbs that also help balance hormones. A combined approach of supporting the liver, enhancing bowel function, replenishing the adrenal glands, and increasing energy levels makes the following supplements invaluable in a natural approach to heavy periods and fibroids.

- Vitamin A
- Vitamin B complex
- Vitamin C and bioflavinoids
- Vitamin D
- Vitamin E
- Omega-3 and omega-6 fatty acids
- Iron-rich formulas
- Magnesium
- Calcium
- Red clover
- Berberis

Progesterone Deficiency

Herbs that support or promote progesterone in perimenopause, treating PMS, and maintaining hormone balance include the following:

- Black cohosh, which relieves PMS depression and insomnia, tonifies or acts like a strengthening or supportive tonic for the uterus, and helps relieve period pain and cramping.
- Dong quai, a Chinese herb that regulates the menstrual cycle, and purifies and tonifies or strengthens the blood.
- Evening primrose oil, which contains gamma-linolenic acid, a precursor to prostaglandins that relieves inflammation and regulates estrogen and progesterone. It is useful for breast tenderness, anxiety, and fatigue.
- Ginger, which is especially useful for the nausea that accompanies severe PMS.
- Red raspberry leaves, a natural source of iron.
- Saint John's wort, useful for treating mild to moderate depression, insomnia, and irritability.
- Vitex (chasteberry), which balances estrogen and progesterone levels and lessens mood swings, anxiety, irritability, and insomnia.
- Wild yam root, which is well known as a source of diosgenin, the natural progesterone precursor. It alleviates inflammation and cramps associated with painful periods and PMS.

Other perimenopausal herbs include:

- Crampbark
- Dandelion root
- Motherwort
- Sarsaparilla root
- Squaw vine
- Yarrow

Cramps

For menstrual cramps, most women use Advil and Motrin medications. The natural approach includes experimenting with dietary restriction the week before the period. Most women benefit by eliminating sugar, alcohol, and meat. Some women may also respond to eliminating dairy or fried foods. The best mineral for helping to squelch menstrual pain is magnesium. The RDA (recommended daily allowance), which is set very low, is about 350 milligrams, but most researchers are suggesting two and three times that amount. Magnesium citrate is the best absorbed and doesn't cause as much of a laxative effect as magnesium oxide. The recommended dosage for the days of painful cramping can be 300 mg taken three or four times per day. However, you may be one of those women who gets constipated before the period, which is a sure sign of magnesium deficiency. Evening primrose oil and fish oils help reduce the inflammation associated with painful periods and are good additions to your supplement protocol.

PMS

Premenstrual syndrome should have no business haunting the lives of women over the age of thirty-five. Unfortunately, it's one of the most common complaints of perimenopausal women. As described in Chapter 4, estrogen dominance plays a dirty trick on our hormones and can trap women in the throes of PMS all month long. When I was in medical practice, I wrote a journal article on PMS because I was having such success with diet, vitamins, minerals, and progesterone suppositories.

Use a chart to keep track of your symptoms to see if they do get worse during the week before your cycle. The symptoms usually occur from ovulation to the period and disappear at the onset of menses. Even if you have estrogen dominance and have symptoms all month long, they will likely be worse before the period. Identifying your symptoms as being cyclical can help to alleviate some of the worry about them.

The most common symptoms of PMS are fluid retention, breast swelling, headaches, mood swings, loss of libido, insomnia, bloating, weight gain, menstrual cramps, fatigue, insomnia, irritability, and anxiety; the first six are symptoms of estrogen dominance. Severe PMS can escalate irritability and mood swings into explosions of anger and rage.

Fluid retention is a big part of PMS, so it's a good idea to avoid foods that contain salt and sugar and therefore exacerbate water retention. That means that chips, sugar, desserts, alcohol, tea, coffee, soft drinks, and processed foods are out. All that miso sauce on sushi can also cause fluid retention—think of the bags under your eyes after a night out at a Japanese restaurant! Try to eat an optimum diet of whole grains, nuts, seeds, vegetables, legumes, fish, and chicken.

The next step is to use vitamin B_6 to decrease fluid buildup; take 100 milligrams, one to three times a day from midcycle to the period. Another deficiency that contributes to premenstrual tension is magnesium; a supplement of 300 milligrams, twice a day, is a good amount to continue all month and can be taken with a calcium supplement of equal strength. The week before the period you can increase these to three a day.

Evening primrose oil is important for relieving breast tenderness and also for painful periods. Take four to six capsules per day. A good all-around vitamin and mineral is also an asset, especially for its B vitamin content to help balance the use of extra B_6.

PMS and Homeopathy

Progesterone deficiency is the main hormonal cause of PMS. Cortisol and progesterone compete for the same receptor sites on cell membranes, with cortisol blocking progesterone activity and leading to estrogen dominance. That's why chronic stress with constantly elevated cortisol can create estrogen dominance and PMS.

With all the triggers for PMS, there is still considerable emotional overlay. Because most women are under such pressure juggling a family and work, additional stress from PMS is often the last straw. Don't let anybody tell you that what you're experiencing is "just an emotional problem," or that an antidepressant or tranquil-izer is all you need.

I add homeopathic medicines to PMS protocols to help create calm in the center of the storm. Homeopathic medicine is diluted and potentized from plants or minerals and prescribed based on the individual's symptoms.

- **Sepia** is for dark-haired women who are angry and irritable and push people away. They feel their uterus is falling and heavy and suffer leg pains prior and during the period but feel much better when they are dancing.
- **Pulsitilla** is for blonde women who are weepy and inconsolable but who also may be changeable; that is, they may appear angry and irritable one moment like a Sepia, and the next minute be in a flood of tears.
- **Nat mur** is a good remedy for women who crave salt. Nat mur is a diluted and potentized form of salt. Women who need this remedy retain a lot of fluid. These women are "shut down"—i.e., they do not want to get emotionally involved with anyone and quite often have suffered a heartache or major grief which keeps them behind a protective barrier. They are often good listeners and try to help others but never get involved.

The potency is 6C, one dose three times a day for seven to ten days before the period for all three homeopathic medicines.

Usually a remedy for PMS is used for three or four menstrual cycles and many symptoms will abate. After that, the remedies are only used as needed.

Dysmenorrhea—Painful Periods

Women with PMS do not necessarily have painful periods. How-ever, when PMS is caused by estrogen dominance an interesting pattern emerges. The endometrial lining of the uterus can extend into the second layer of the uterus, called the adenomyosis, the muscle wall. When the lining of the uterus sheds during menses, some of the blood will become temporarily trapped in the muscle wall and cause pain and inflammation. Anti-inflammatory pills may lessen symptoms but the real cause is low levels of progesterone. Once that imbalance is resolved, the uterine lining builds with estrogen and matures with progesterone and sheds without interfering with the muscular wall.

Treatment for Candida albicans

The following is a brief outline of major steps in Candida treatment. Please see the late Dr. William Crook's work at *www.yeast connection.com* for more detailed shopping lists and recipes for overcoming Candida. I first met Dr. Crook in 1986 on a 90-minute television talk show in Toronto, Canada. The topic was candidiasis, and we were swamped with calls from interested viewers. The station sent me a thank-you letter with the startling statistic that almost 80,000 people called into the show that evening. I'm now a medical advisor to yeastconnection.com, a site run by the late Dr. Crook's daughter, Elizabeth Crook. I can't emphasize enough how important a condition candidiasis is and how necessary it is to follow a comprehensive treatment program. Just taking an antifungal drug won't be enough. A program should include the following elements:

DIET
Emphasize a diet rich in free-range and organic meats, fish, chicken, eggs, seeds and nuts, vegetables, and oils. Avoid sugars, carbohydrate-rich foods, and fermented products such as vinegars and preserved meats to starve the yeast. Eat plenty of garlic, onions, and chives, which have antifungal properties. Use coconut oil for its beneficial medium-chain fatty acids that suppress yeast.

SUPPLEMENTS

Probiotics are friendly bacteria that help you keep a natural, healthy balance of microorganisms in your digestive tract. To be effective, it's best if they are enteric-coated; this helps to bypass the harsh stomach acid and deliver at least 1 billion live organisms to the intestines.

DIGESTIVE ENZYMES

These enzymes help maintain a natural, healthy digestion. Most good products contain several enzymes to promote optimal digestion. It's also helpful to include phytonutrients, or plant nutrients from herbs such as peppermint to help maintain and calm an upset stomach.

HERBS AND NUTRIENTS

Herbs and nutrients that can be used to inhibit the growth of Candida albicans include caprylic acid, Pau d'Arco, oregano oil, black walnut, grapefruit seed extract, garlic, beta carotene, and biotin.

VITAMINS AND MINERALS

Taking a good-quality daily multivitamin and mineral supplement helps supply your body with the nutrients it needs to help you regain your health. Good calcium, magnesium, and vitamin D supplements are also essential to optimal health, especially for women.

AVOID EXPOSURE TO CHEMICALS

Paints, household cleaners, perfumes, and scents may cause allergic reactions. Chemical sensitivities are very common in people with yeast overgrowth.

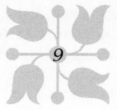

9

Menopause: Was It Ever a Disease?

MENOPAUSE IS A NATURAL OCCURRENCE. It happens to every woman who lives long enough to "enjoy" this stage of life, and it's happening to the more than two million women entering menopause every year in America. However, unnatural circumstances can make menopause a difficult time that must be endured rather than enjoyed! Before we get to that, let's look at what menopause is really about.

✻ True Menopause

Menopause is defined as one year without periods. It's a retrospective diagnosis. You look back and notice that you haven't marked any red slashes in your calendar for twelve months. In that case, you're one of the lucky ones if your periods just quietly slipped off into the sunset. Most books on menopause say the average age is fifty-one. However, the range can be from age forty to sixty.

There's not much more to be said about menopause. That's why most books and articles on the topic go on to describe menopausal symptoms, and how to avoid them and the increased risk of heart disease and osteoporosis that come with this life change. I'll do the same here, but first a word on how society's view of menopause has changed in the past decade.

You've Come a Long Way, Baby

Years ago, people didn't really talk about menopause. It's only in the last decade that baby boomers have made menopause a popular topic. Boomers are breaking tradition on all fronts, and age isn't what it used to be. When my mother was fifty-five she wouldn't dream of rollerblading on the Venice boardwalk or staying up all night at a rock concert. It just wasn't done. Whereas at fifty-five I do just that! There are no restrictions—physically, mentally, or culturally—on what women can do.

The only positive image of menopause when I was growing up was the Wise Crone figure. Today, most women won't settle for that. The wisdom, yes, but not the crone. Sure, the wrinkles and the sagging are going to come and I'm not a proponent of plastic surgery, but the power of diet, supplements, and exercise is phenomenal. Today the Wise Crone can be wrapped up in Warrior leather or silk and lace. Save the long woolen dresses for a few more decades!

Stopping the Clock

When I first wrote about menopause in 1999, I spoke about it as a time when women feel relieved from the burden of childbearing and child rearing. Even that's debatable these days. After all, many women are waiting until the imaginary clock stops at age forty to have their first child. That means even more menopausal stress for a whole generation of business-mothers when they enter menopause. Another worry is that late pregnancies are probably a trigger for early menopause, especially if getting pregnant requires fertility drugs. This means that for some women menopause will be closer to forty-five than fifty.

I also wrote that menopause is "a time for a woman to grow spiritually and intellectually and take her place as a 'wise woman' in the community, as in China, Japan, South Africa, and among Native Americans." I still believe in those words, but I am afraid it's not going to be easy for menopausal moms to find any time to sit and meditate, with their kids still demanding constant attention.

Menopausal Fears

Whether bringing up preteens or babysitting the grandchildren, menopause for many women becomes a time of unnecessary fear and uncertainty. Drug companies make women fear osteoporosis and aging. Society makes women afraid of growing old and forgotten.

The unnatural circumstances that make for a difficult menopause have already been identified throughout the book. Xenoestrogens in our air, food, and water, adrenal depletion, hypothyroidism, overgrowth of Candida albicans, and the overuse of drugs can all lead to hormone imbalance. These unnatural circumstances also include the way menopause has been viewed by the medical profession as a disease in need of treatment. In medical school, menopause was said to be primarily a condition caused by a deficiency of estrogen. I was very fortunate, however, to be trained at a time when even the staunchest supporter of ERT was cowed by the incontrovertible reports that estrogen causes uterine cancer.

Advertising Menopause

Dr. Robert A. Wilson wrote *Feminine Forever* before the moratorium in the mid-1970s on ERT. But that embargo lasted only a few years before the barrage of promotion for HRT, a combination of synthetic estrogen and synthetic progesterone, which was supposed to prevent uterine cancer. Both doctors and drug advertisers for the last several decades have been forcing women to make a choice between taking synthetic hormones with the possible consequences of getting cancer versus not taking synthetic hormones and getting heart disease or osteoporosis. We now know that HRT does not prevent heart disease and is only somewhat useful in preventing osteoporosis, plus it has many side effects.

Menopausal Complaints

Every woman past forty-five knows that many doctors seem to toss away their responsibility to diagnose women's symptoms past a certain age. The magic number seems to be forty-five when doctors begin to tell their female patients that all their symptoms must be due to menopause or aging. If you resist, they just say, "You can't expect to stay twenty-nine forever."

Know Thyself

Menopause gives women a definable time to look at life and health and make choices. By knowing the difference between symptoms of menopause and symptoms of aging you can, at the very least, avoid unnecessary over-the-counter and prescription drugs. And whether the symptoms are due to aging or menopause, there are many commonsense and natural solutions that you can use before turning to medication. Statistics on drug use in seniors shows an average use of between eight and ten different prescription medications each year.

Realizing that menopause is not a disease and that you can be healthy your whole life empowers you to take charge of your health. Let's look at the symptoms of menopause, what causes them, and why we fear them. The main ones of concern are hot flashes, weight gain, vaginal dryness, mood swings, loss of energy, and skin and hair changes. Longer-range concerns include osteoporosis, and heart and vascular disease. The therapeutic approaches to these conditions are found in Chapters 11 to 13.

✖ Menopause Power Surges

One inspired patient of mine, who turned red from her scalp to her chest several times a day with her hot flashes, handed out niacin tablets to her unsympathetic family. She was tired of their jokes about her beet-red face and dripping perspiration. Vitamin B_3 is now used in prescription medications to lower cholesterol. As niacin, but not niacinamide, it causes a strong prickly heat flush over the whole body that is much like a hot flash. The sensation occurs mainly in sun-exposed areas. Fifty to 100 milligrams will do the trick.

Hot Flashes

Is it hot flushes or hot flashes? A hot flash is more descriptive of the onset of this menopausal event. A sudden sense of heat occurs, mostly in the face and neck and also the upper chest, then the red flush comes like a severe blush from a major embarrassment. Hot flashes in bed can cause drenching sweats that have you up at night changing nighties and sheets. The terms hot flash and hot flush are used quite interchangeably in most texts and there is usually no attempt to differentiate. Either way they are very common, occurring in up to 85 percent of women during their menopause.

Beyond the heat, the red flush, and the sweating, hot flashes may be associated with a rapid heartbeat, nausea, dizziness, anxiety, headache, weakness, or a feeling of suffocation. Some texts talk about an "aura" or an uneasiness that precedes the hot flash, as though the lights dim, the scary music comes, and suddenly you're flashing. When I went into menopause very suddenly one year when I was under massive stress, I experienced a symptom I had never heard before. My "aura" was an incredible sense of impending doom that would descend on my body just before a hot flash burnt me to a crisp and then drenched me in sweat, followed by a chilling clamminess.

What Causes Hot Flashes?

In medical school I was taught that hot flashes occur because of low estrogen levels. But now I know that women have hot flashes in perimenopause, when estrogen levels are high, as well as long after menopause when they are very low. While most experts readily agree that we really don't know exactly what causes hot flashes, we do know that it is a "vasomotor reaction" to hormonal shifts. Vaso-motor reaction means a nerve and muscle reaction that occurs in blood vessels, causing them to constrict or dilate.

Apparently FSH, which stimulated a developing egg and LH (luteinizing hormone) and which stimulates ripening follicles in the ovary to produce estrogen, can be elevated when hot flashes occur. Both these hormones become elevated with menopause. Research shows that neurotransmitters and erratic hormones can cause blood vessels near the surface of the skin, especially in the head, neck and chest, to become dilated, which creates heat, blushing, and sweat-ing. Hormonal surges of cortisol can also create hot flashes.

The medical experts at breastcancer.org give the following expla-nation for hot flashes. They say the hypothalamus is in charge of regulating estrogen levels. It presides over body temperature, appe-tite, and sleep cycles as well as sex hormones. A diminished level of estrogen triggers the hypothalamus, which somehow confuses its thermostat and reads the message that the body is too hot. In order to get the body to sweat and therefore cool off, a dizzying array of signals are sent out that leads to the release of the adrenal hormone epinephrine (thus the feeling of impending doom) and other hormones that increase the heart rate, circulate more blood, dilate blood vessels on the skin, and cause the release of sweat from glands close to the skin. All these actions are designed to cool the skin, resulting in hot flashes and severe sweats. But in the meantime, these confused messages cause heat. Research shows a rise of skin temperature by as much as six degrees during a hot flash, which causes you to sweat—and then you are left in a puddle.

Avoiding Flash Triggers

Research tells us that our core temperature goes up just before a hot flash. That means turn up the air conditioning and don't allow yourself to get overheated. For me, I couldn't take my hot, Epsom salt baths for years and had to swear off the saunas that I also loved.

Track down other triggers that make you flash. Get a bright red notebook and jot down what you are eating, wearing, and stressing about when you get your hot flashes. Also give them a score—from 1 for fuzzy (as in warm and fuzzy) up to 10 for deadly, as in dynamite. Finding names for your flashes can help to distract you from the abuse they inflict on you. One hot flash trigger that took me time to identify was the cinnamon I put on my Crock-Pot cereal in the morning. (More about Crock-Pot cereal in Chapter 11.) Cinnamon is a hot spice, and it was revving me up, increasing the heat in my body and stimulating more hot flashes. Most spicy foods can do the same. Other triggers include sugar, smoking, alcohol, and caffeine (found in coffee, chocolate, diet pills, or pain pills).

What's Stress Got to Do with It?

As we've said, stress has a tremendous impact on everything about our health. And stressing is the worst trigger for flashes. For some women, hot flashes work like aversion therapy to stop stressful behavior. I know for me they did. Every time I took a nosedive into some primal fear or worry I'd trigger a hot flash, so I just don't go there anymore! Stress from overwork and rushing can also increase hot flashes. Look at them as a reason to slow down and take some time for yourself.

Now that you know what your triggers are, here are some survival tips.

- Wear layers of clothing, in natural fibers, so you can peel them off when necessary. Synthetics do not allow the skin to breathe.
- Forget about turtleneck sweaters.
- Keep a fan handy.
- Keep ice water nearby—either throw it over yourself or take a long drink to cool your skin and your core temperature!
- Deep breathing can reduce hot flashes by about 40 percent.
- Wear cotton to bed and use cotton sheets—you may not need a blanket!
- Take a cool shower at bedtime.

Exercise Your Flashes Away

Exercise is beneficial for more than just hot flashes and more than just menopause. It should be part of your daily routine already, but if it's not, here are the reasons why you need to begin: It can reduce hot flashes, help you lose weight, condition your muscles, improve bone density, prevent heart disease, lower cholesterol, balance moods by increasing endorphins, reduce insomnia, decrease fatigue, increase sexual desire, and improve confidence.

Stress Busters

Here are some more ways to relieve stress:

- Sleep!—at least seven hours a night
- Relaxation exercises
- Deep breathing
- Meditation
- Yoga
- Visualization
- Tai Chi
- Body work—deep tissue massage, craniosacral therapy, lymphatic massage
- Biofeedback
- Self-hypnosis

Sleep

An additional word about sleep—it's the most important stress buster of all. We all know what sleepless nights do to us. It's the same for inadequate sleep. If you are trying to make your life work by cutting back on sleep, you are putting too much stress on your body. During sleep is when your body is able to repair and restore. If you can't sleep because of menopause symptoms, I'll give you lots of advice in Chapters 11 and 12. If you have always had a sleep problem you can take magnesium, calcium, and vitamin B complex and use herbal combinations of hops, valerian, skullcap, Saint Johns wort, chamomile, and passion flower. A homeopathic medicine called Gelsemium can be used for insomnia due to worry. If you wake up at night and can't get back to sleep because you can't stop thinking about something or worrying, take a few pellets of Gelsemium 6X under your tongue.

Drugs for Hot Flashes

In Chapters 11 and 12 we'll talk about the dietary and supplement approach to treating hot flashes and in Chapter 13 address the use of bioidentical hormones as a possible safer solution than synthetic HRT. I was surprised to find that as an alternative to synthetic ERT, doctors are prescribing a new breed of antidepressants such as Effexor for hot flashes and night sweats. They are not of the Prozac variety, but they do seem to have a high rate of side effects. However if your symptoms are severe enough, a trial of this drug might be warranted. Even so, Effexor only seems to reduce the symptoms of hot flashes by about 60 percent.

Here is a list of Effexor side effects and the percentage of people experiencing each effect.

- Nausea: 37%
- Headache: 25%
- Sleepiness: 23%
- Dry mouth: 22%
- Dizziness: 19%
- Insomnia: 18%
- Constipation: 15%
- Nervousness: 13%
- Raised blood pressure: 13%
- Fatigue: 12%
- Sweating: 12%

Vaginal Dryness

Sex shouldn't be painful, but it is with vaginal dryness. Washing the urogenital area with too much soap dries the skin out even more, so that when you go to the bathroom, urine burns, and when you wipe, it hurts. The mucus cells that line the vagina are directly stimulated by estrogen, making them fat and juicy. As estrogen levels diminish, that layer of lubricating cells is replaced with ones that are flat and dry as paper. All those rumors that you've been hearing that sex and orgasm stimulates hormones are true. Go ahead and try it out, whether you have a partner or not, and you'll see the benefits.

A healthy vaginal lining is not just for lubrication but is also a protective layer. When that's gone, the dryness can lead to minor abrasions from the trauma of intercourse or even from a harsh washing or wiping of the genitals. These tiny tears can be invaded by bacteria and yeast causing an irritating infection.

We'll be talking more about the herbal treatment of menopause in Chapter 12. Briefly, however, studies have shown that in some women, taking black cohosh, as part of a menopausal supplement program, can help correct vaginal dryness. Vitamin E, orally, with 400 IU once or twice a day can also be useful. Some women open up a capsule and insert the oil into the vaginal opening.

Estrogen is what the vagina wants, but many women are leery of using any estrogen products. However studies do show that it is the safest way to keep the vaginal tissues alive and not produce elevated blood levels of estrogen and is without side effects.[30] I personally use estriol vaginal cream, an amount the size of the tip of my little finger twice a week, and it does the trick. Estriol cream is only available on prescription; the dosage is usually 0.5mg/gram, one gram per day for seven days when starting treatment, then one gram per week on a continuous basis. You will usually notice the difference within two weeks.

The best stimulant for a healthy vagina is the practice of regular sexual activity, so once you get dryness under control you can enjoy sex more. Sexual arousal leads to vaginal lubrication; that's another function of those estrogen-craving vaginal cells. In turn, the moisture heals the vaginal tissues. In a younger woman it may only take thirty seconds to a minute of foreplay to produce enough lubricating mucus for painless intercourse. In an older woman, however, it may take several minutes. Therefore, put more emphasis on foreplay. Water-soluble lubricants such as K-Y jelly can be used to help with lubrication. But not with condoms, as there is a chemical ingredient in K-Y jelly that causes holes to develop in latex!

I have a great concern about the widespread use of Viagra in older men. I'm afraid they may get a bit carried away with their "new toy" and not wait for their partner to be ready for intercourse. I've heard numerous reports—it's not front-page news—about tears, abrasions, and infections in older women having sex with Viagra-driven men. Maybe there's a reason why Mr. Limp is the way he is. Both partners need to take time with foreplay as we age.

Vaginitis

Up to 50 percent of chronic vaginal infections are due to yeast. The diagnosis can often be made by observing a white, cheesy discharge with a "yeasty" odor. Women are more susceptible if they are on the BCP, ERT, or HRT, have a diet high in sugar and processed foods, or drink alcohol.

In my experience, a vaginal swab can be negative for yeast almost 50 percent of the time. This may occur because labs are focused on finding bacteria, and therefore the "growing media" that is used to "culture" throat, rectal, and vaginal swabs is suited more to bacteria than yeast.

A bacterial vaginitis can usually by diagnosed by a swab. The most common ones are Gardnerella, Strep, or Hemophilus. If the swab is positive but there are no signs of systemic infection—no pain on internal pelvic exam, no fever or chills—the treatment can be with a simple betadine or boric acid douche. If the bacterial infection is gonorrhea or chlamydia, then the treatment is with oral antibiotics. Remember to take lactobacillis acidophilus capsules to prevent yeast infection when you take an antibiotic but take them several hours away from each other.

For a yeast infection here are some useful tips:

- Avoid tight synthetic undergarments and pants.
- Wear loose cotton underwear, which may have to be boiled, microwaved, or ironed to kill all the yeast spores!
- Avoid acidifying spermicides, which can irritate the vagina and encourage yeast overgrowth.
- Don't wipe with scented or dyed toilet paper and don't use scented or deodorized pads or tampons.
- If you are still menstruating, alternate between pads and tampons.
- Use a condom to be sure your partner is not passing yeast back to you during intercourse.
- Natural douches include one tablespoon of baking soda in a pint of water; two tablespoons of acidophilus or yogurt in a pint of water; one tablespoon of vinegar in a pint of water; or one teaspoon (that's *teaspoon*) of boric acid in a pint of water. You should douche twice a day, morning and night, for five days.

Treatment for simple yeast vaginitis can often be accomplished with a simple douche. In some cases this may be enough to provide symptomatic relief. If vaginitis persists, it must be treated on a broader scale with diet: acidophilus by mouth, acidophilus mixed with yogurt to make a paste that can be used vaginally, and sometimes oral antifungal medications.

Vaginal candidiasis is very common, especially if you eat sugar on a daily basis. Working with yeastconnection.com, I have heard the most horrendous stories about mistreated vaginal candidiasis. The problem is that most doctors don't understand that the treatment is not just a vaginal antifungal suppository or an oral antifungal pill. Sugar and alcohol, and even wheat and dairy, have the ability to stimulate the growth of Candida in the intestines and in the vagina. See the section on Candida albicans in Chapter 8 for an overview of the full treatment protocol, and use yeastconnection. com as your Candida resource.

Incontinence

Another irritating symptom of a dry vagina is more frequent trips to the bathroom. As if you aren't already going every hour on the hour! With thinning tissues in the genitourinary area this is a common symptom. It's also blamed on previous pregnancies resulting in a falling pelvic floor. Sounds like a construction site gone wrong, and not something you want to hear about. However, you can do something about a falling pelvic floor; see the description of Kegel exercises just below.

For dry vagina, I have tried the obvious things. I always use a natural pH soap, such as castile, in the vaginal area; I always wear cotton underwear. I did find that tight pants were irritating, and I was going to the bathroom far too much. At first, I used a natural vaginal lubricant and tried progesterone creams. For me personally, I couldn't find anything natural that would make those cells plump up. I went to my doctor and had an estrogen index done on my Pap test, which found that my estrogen-dependent vaginal cells were indeed diminishing rapidly, so I was given a prescription for estriol vaginal cream. In the beginning I used it every day for one week, now I just apply a tiny amount twice a week. It was amazing how quickly the vaginal lining came back to life and I even have less frequent urination.

Some tips for avoiding incontinence:

- Avoid alcohol, which is a great irritant to the bladder sphincter.
- Avoid caffeine, which causes increased urination (it's found in colas, chocolate, pain medication, and diet pills).

- Don't smoke, as it causes irritation of the bladder, and "smoker's cough" can cause bladder leaking when the whole body goes into reflex spasm from the cough.
- Lose weight.
- Avoid constipation.

Kegel Exercises

While searching for relief of my urinary frequency I was reminded of Kegel exercises. Although they are used mainly for urinary incontinence, they can also be extremely helpful in strengthening the muscles around the urethra and vagina. They can be of benefit to your sex life as well. Kegel is the name of a pelvic floor exercise; it's named after Dr. Arnold Kegel, who invented it. These muscles are attached to the pelvic bone and act like a hammock, holding in your pelvic organs. To isolate these muscles, try stopping and starting the flow of urine. Involuntary leakage of urine (urinary incontinence) is the bane of many of us who've reached our forties—and it often affects younger women, too. Decreasing levels of estrogen can weaken the muscles that have control over the urethra (the tube carrying urine from the bladder to the outside of the body). Other factors, such as weight gain as we get older, can make incontinence worse.

Here are the how-to's for Kegel exercises:

STEP 1

Locate the muscles on your pelvic floor by contracting the muscles around your urethra as if you're trying to hold back the flow of urine. You may have to put your finger in your vagina to practice the proper contraction. Then, practice with a partially full bladder. Start and stop the flow several times. Stopping the flow tightens the pelvic floor while starting the flow relaxes it. Now you can move on to Step 2.

STEP 2

Contract and release the pelvic floor muscles quickly and firmly. Use your finger in the vagina again to practice. Keep everything else relaxed except the muscles right around the vagina. Don't become tense and hold your breath. You can do the exercises with your knees together (lying or sitting); start with two five-minute sessions per day. Squeeze for a count of four and relax for a count of four.

STEP 3

Repeat Step 2, but this time with your knees apart and squeeze for a count of eight and then relax for a count of eight. Repeat this for five minutes two times a day.

STEP 4

Do the "elevator exercise" by imagining your pelvic floor is an elevator. Contract the muscles upward from the first floor to the fifth floor, stopping at each floor and getting tighter as you go higher. Then, release downward, releasing tension as you go down. Get further control over your pelvic floor muscles by pushing them down "to the basement." Practice this with your bladder empty.

STEP 5

Do daily Kegel practice sessions in which you firmly and quickly contract and release your pelvic floor muscles ten times a session, five to ten times daily. Then do the elevator exercise in which you work up to the tenth floor. Do this five times a session at least three times a day. Then add the "basement" level to the elevator. Finally, tense from front to back, then release back to front. Do this five times a day, three times day.

STEP 6

Once you are through the learning phase, you achieve good muscle tone with just five minutes twice a day. Doing them in bed in the morning and at night works for some women. When you have achieved your goal you can maintain muscle tone with just five minutes three times a week.

Bladder Infection

The lower lining of the urethra at the end of the bladder can also be affected by lack of estrogen. Cells in this region produce mucus but only grow and produce under the direction of estrogen. An irritated urethra is subject to bacterial infections that can travel into the bladder. A minor bladder infection might not just produce frequent urination but be a constant drain on the immune system as well.

The most common cause of bladder infections in women tends to be from intercourse. During intercourse, the positioning of the penis can be such that the urethra is trapped and irritated. This will cause the urethra to swell. There can be bacteria near the urethra, which can migrate from the rectal area. The urethral inflammation and swelling provides an ideal environment for bacteria to grow.

To avoid bladder infections after intercourse, take care to not create this jamming action with the penis that traps the urethra; just pull back an inch or so if this is happening. Wash before and after intercourse with a neutral pH soap and also urinate before and after intercourse to wash bacteria out of the urethra.

If bladder symptoms begin—frequent urination, burning, and pressure—it is important to take a clean urine sample to your doctor so that she or he may have it tested for bacterial overgrowth. Be sure to wash well before urinating and keep your pubic hairs from touching the urine stream. Void a small amount of urine first into the toilet to flush out bacteria that may just be resting outside the urethra, then fill the specimen jar. While waiting for results of your urine test there are several natural treatments that you can use.

- Drink ½ to ¼ teaspoon of baking soda in one glass of water every thirty minutes—this can help make the urine less acidic and therefore burn less. (Avoid if you have a heart condition.)
- Avoid tea and coffee.
- Take parsley or chamomile tea, four cups per day.
- Take Uva ursi capsules, two capsules three times per day.
- Take cranberry concentrate capsules, six to eight per day.
- Drink unsweetened cranberry juice.
- Drink lots of water, as it's the key to flushing out bacteria.
- Homeopathic Cantharis or Causticum in the 6C or 30C potency taken every hour can be helpful.
- For postcoital irritation, Homeopathic Staphasagria 6C or 30C can be taken every hour.
- Avoid tight synthetic undergarments or pants, wear loose cotton underwear, and avoid scented tampons and pads and even colored toilet paper.
- After a bowel movement, wipe from front to back to avoid pulling bowel bacteria into the vaginal and urethral area.

Sexual Satisfaction

Now that we have vaginal dryness, incontinence, and urogenital infections under control, we can start thinking about sex. It is possible that sex takes a back seat—oops, wrong metaphor—it's possible that sex loses its zing because of all the problems that arise when there isn't enough estrogen to keep the vagina lubricated. I can see why women got on the estrogen bandwagon to relieve themselves of this major menopausal problem.

Suzanne Somers is right: Menopause can be the sexy years for many women. Especially if your kids are off on their own, you and your partner now have the freedom to be together and make up for all those nights lost while raising a family. Estriol vaginal cream may be all you need, along with diet and natural supplements to achieve the sexy years. We'll talk more about these supplements in Chapter 12 and also about Suzanne's bioidentical hormones in Chapter 13.

✄ Heart Palpitations

Since the adrenal glands are called into play as the sex hormones decline, you can have episodes of adrenal surges that you may not notice, except that the adrenaline can trigger heart palpitations. If you are experiencing heart palpitations, it's important to see your doctor. Heart disease does affect as many women as men, but we don't seem to have the same dramatic symptoms that everyone identifies with a heart attack. Instead of severe chest pain, sweating, and severe shortness of breath, women may feel breathless without chest pain; feel nauseated and clammy; feel fatigued, weak, and dizzy; have pain in the jaw, neck, shoulders, upper back, and chest; and feel very anxious.

If you have heart palpitations, it's time to put away your coffee cup. Caffeine is the most common cause of this condition. Magnesium is a very common mineral deficiency in anyone having heart palpitations. I used to have heart palpitations, but not after I increased my daily dose of magnesium. It's also important to take equal amounts of calcium and magnesium. We take far too much calcium compared to magnesium, mostly because we've been told that calcium is the most important mineral for bone health, but magnesium is just as crucial for both bone and heart health.

Angina and Atherosclerosis

Angina is a condition of aging blood vessels. There have been decades of speculation that estrogen is protective against heart disease. Women before the age of menopause have a lower incidence of heart disease than they do after menopause when estrogen is lower.

However, the WHI study of both HRT and ERT informs us that at least synthetic estrogen and progestins are not protective of the heart and should not be prescribed for this reason.

Angina is a pain in the chest or shoulder; it is a reaction to the coronary blood vessels either going into spasm or being blocked by cholesterol plaque. The pain symptom usually occurs on exertion and should be thoroughly investigated by a medical doctor.

I suspect that many women have heart symptoms due to magnesium deficiency. When I researched my book on magnesium (*The Miracle of Magnesium*, Ballantine, 2003), I found that women generally seem to have lower magnesium levels than men. It would be interesting to do a study on the amount of plaque in the arteries of women who have heart disease. The lower the plaque, the more evidence of magnesium as the underlying cause.

An optimum diet, exercise, weight loss, no smoking, and minimum alcohol are all part of a healthy heart protocol. Supplements that help heal the heart include.

- Vitamin C: 1,000 mg per day as an antioxidant
- Vitamin E: as mixed tocopherols and tocotrienols: 400–800 units per day as an antioxidant
- Magnesium: 300 mg, three times per day for heart spasms and palpitations
- B complex: 50 mg to calm the nervous system, one or two per day
- A good multiple vitamin and mineral
- Garlic, hawthorn berry herbal tinctures: 5 to 10 drops in four ounces of water three times a day

An alternative, but invasive, method for treating atherosclerosis, angina, and heart disease is chelation therapy. An intravenous injection of a mineral binding agent removes the mineral/cholesterol plaque from the artery walls, and in numerous studies this has proven beneficial in reversing heart disease. This procedure should be done by a medical professional who has had special training and certification with the American Board of Chelation Therapy or the American College of Advancement in Medicine.

> *American Board of Chelation Therapy*
> 1407-B North Wells St.
> Chicago, IL 60610
> 800-356-2228

> *American College of Advancement in Medicine*
> 23121 Verdugo Dr., Suite 204
> Laguna Hills, CA 92653
> 714-583-7666
> 800-532-3688

Hair Loss

Losing hair on the head and gaining it on the chin doesn't seem to be a fair tradeoff. Hair loss occurring at menopause is often due to over-production of dihydrotestosterone that affects the hair follicle. This produces male-pattern baldness in women. Stress makes the process worse. As the stress hormones are revved up in the adrenal glands, that action also triggers the production of more male hormones. A diet high in refined carbohydrates and excess body fat only makes things worse by further stimulating male hormone production. De-stressing, with the optimum diet outlined in Chapter 11, and adrenal support, as noted in Chapter 5, can help to reverse the imbalance of hormones. That's what *Hormone Balance* is all about, naturally—achieving balance among your hormones.

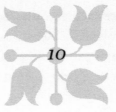

10

Baby Boomers Losing Bone

YEARS AGO I LEARNED OF a study by a woman anthropologist who measured the bone densities of a group of strong young South American women. They effortlessly carried enormous jars overflowing with water on their head up and down treacherous trails. Decades later the same anthropologist went back to the same village and found the same women, older, grayer, but still effortlessly carrying those same jars. Their bone density tests showed that their bones were thinning, just as our bones do. However, lifting and carrying those heavy jars kept their muscles, tendons, and cartilage strong, and these older women did not break bones or show symptoms of osteoporosis. It always made me wonder how much our bone density tests correlate with actual disease.

Osteoporosis Overview

Osteoporosis has become a dreaded aspect of menopause. We hear about it constantly in the media, from our doctors, and from our friends. The National Osteoporosis Foundation calls it a "major public threat for an estimated 44 million Americans." They estimate that, as of June 2004, ten million individuals in the United States already have the disease and almost thirty-four million more have low bone mass, placing them at increased risk for osteoporosis. One in every two women will have an osteoporosis-related fracture sometime in their life. Every year there are more than 1.5 million fractures; the estimated direct cost for hospitalization and nursing home care in 2001 was $17 billion—an amazing $47 million every day!

Most women don't know they have osteoporosis until they sustain a fracture, often from a relatively minor incident. Vertebrae are the first to go, as they become porous, weaken, and then suddenly collapse, leaving the characteristic stooped posture and loss of height we see in the elderly. What makes menopause the target of osteoporosis is that women can lose up to 20 percent of their bone mass in the five to seven years following menopause. If the bones are thin to start with, then there is an increased risk of osteoporosis and fractures.

Porous bone defines the condition. We are told that, remarkably, by our early twenties, we have built up about 98 percent of our bone mass. From then on it's a matter of remodeling as minerals are added and subtracted from bone. When more minerals are broken down from bone than replaced, the bones become thin. For example, during pregnancy, if you don't take enough calcium, magnesium, zinc, copper, and boron, your bones are scavenged for these minerals to create the skeletal structure of your growing child. However, there is a natural fail-safe for this loss. Calcitonin, a hormone that helps keep bone from breaking down, is increased during pregnancy to replace the losses due to the new baby.

As a teenager, if you drink soda every day—phosphorus in the drink leaches minerals, especially calcium, from bone—you may have thinner bones going into adulthood. Cigarette smoking and alcohol and even eating too much sugar can also take their toll on bone. However, exercising and taking calcium and magnesium can make your bones dense and solid, so you can afford to lose some bone mass around menopause.

The History of Osteoporosis

It turns out that osteoporosis does not have a history. It appears to be a new disease. Is it another condition caused by our "civilized" lifestyle? Whenever I write about a disease, I consult my 1892 "Practical Home Physician" to get a sense of the evolution of the condition. In its 1,300 pages, however, there is no mention of osteoporosis. Under fractures, there is a listing of every bone in the body and how to set it and treat it. For the entry on hip fracture, the following is written: "The hip bone itself is very strong and well protected; hence it is seldom broken. The fracture of the bone is not an especially serious injury, and recovery may occur without deformity or subsequent difficulty."

The authors of this passage are not concerned about millions of hip fractures or brittle bones that shatter on the least impact. Some researchers believe that it's not even a fall that causes most of the broken bones; instead, the hip or thigh bone just cracks from the pressure of walking and this is what causes the fall. One hundred years ago, bones seemed to be much stronger. It is very important that we identify what has happened since then to make osteoporosis so prevalent.

It's Not All about Calcium

Preventing osteoporosis actually begins in the womb! Most doctors agree that you have to build strong bones during childhood and adolescence as a defense against osteoporosis, but you must begin much earlier. The medical emphasis on calcium and estrogen as the treatments for osteoporosis is very limited. Bones are not just made of calcium. If they were, they would be very brittle and breaking all the time. In fact, according to bone expert Dr. Susan Brown, bone requires eighteen nutrients for proper growth. The emphasis on calcium as the only treatment for osteoporosis may actually be one reason why they are breaking all the time.

Chronically low intake of calcium, magnesium, vitamin D, boron, and vitamins K, B_{12}, B_6, and folic acid lead to osteoporosis. Chronically high intake of protein, sodium chloride, alcohol, and caffeine adversely affect bone health.[31] It appears that the typical Western diet (high in protein and salt and in refined, processed foods), lack of exercise, and lack of supplemental nutrient intake contributes to the epidemic of osteoporosis. I consider osteoporosis to be another lifestyle condition, much like hypertension or obesity, which is amenable to the right diet and supplements.

What Makes Up Bone

Bone is a living tissue made up of organic and inorganic material. The organic matrix is like a web to which minerals adhere and form hard bones. This organic part makes up about 35 percent of bone. It is formed from tough collagen fibers; two types of cells—osteoblasts, which are bone-forming cells, and osteoclasts, the bone-absorbing cells; and nerves, blood vessels, and pain receptors. The main mineral of bone is calcium. That's why most doctors advise calcium supplements to prevent osteoporosis. However, along with calcium there are phosphate, magnesium, sodium, potassium, zinc, manganese, and molybdenum.

There is rapid turnover of bone constituents—97 percent of the body's calcium is found in bones and teeth, and when it is required in other parts of the body osteoclasts release it. The same can be said for magnesium—65 percent of the body's magnesium is stored in bones and teeth. Most people imagine that bone is just a dead tissue to which we can add some calcium to make it stronger. Nothing could be further from the truth. Bone is constantly changing, being remodeled, and, if we give it the right building blocks, improving. I've read that our entire skeleton is remodeled every five years. To me that's great news. It means we have a chance to make a whole new skeleton in the next five years. With the right diet, nutrients, and exercise we can make it much stronger and much healthier.

⚘ Osteoporosis Risk Factors

The risk factors for osteoporosis are varied. The first group includes factors over which we have little control.

- Having abnormal bone density
- Having a history of fracture in mother or sister
- Being female
- Being thin and/or having a small frame
- Being of Northern European ancestry
- Being light-haired and light-skinned
- Being at an advanced age
- Having a family history of osteoporosis
- Having estrogen deficiency as a result of menopause, especially early or surgically induced
- Having an abnormal absence of menstrual periods (amenorrhea)

The next group of risk factors consists of ones that we can control. Some of them are well-known risks, but magnesium deficiency and soda pop intake will not appear in medical texts about osteoporosis.

- Low lifetime calcium intake
- Low intake of magnesium

- Regular use of antacids containing aluminum
- Regular intake of soda pop
- Regular use of coffee
- Vitamin D deficiency—very common in northern climates
- Long history of a poor diet
- Use of certain medications, such as corticosteroids and anti-convulsants
- Presence of certain chronic medical conditions—anorexia, kidney disease, liver disease
- Presence of periodontal disease
- An inactive lifestyle
- Current cigarette smoking
- Excessive use of alcohol

The third list is from Annemarie Colbin's book *Food and Our Bones*. She says that, based on her lifelong experience with food and lifestyle, she has come to the conclusion that the following have a direct *negative* impact on our bones. It's a very "proactive" list—it digs at the very foundation of osteoporosis and gives us clues to help us make a change in how we view osteoporosis and how we can both prevent and treat it.

- Eating a high proportion of animal protein together with flour products and sweets
- Eating a high proportion of nightshade vegetables (potatoes, tomatoes, eggplant, peppers)
- Not eating enough vegetables
- Not including enough good-quality fats in the diet
- Not including enough protein in the diet

In the treatment section, I will go over a comprehensive diet, supplement, and exercise program for osteoporosis. As you can see from the second list, physical inactivity is a factor in thinning bones.

What you may not know is that during the first weightless space flights, astronauts lost both bone mass and muscle mass as a direct result of inactivity. Our structure demands movement in order to stay strong. How you move it and how often you move it are both important. For example, if you walk with your feet turned out you change the natural anatomical alignment of your leg in relation to your hip. After a few million steps with the wrong alignment, your hip joint is going to suffer. Based on the uneven pressure on the joint, one side will build up more bone and the other side will weaken.

✴ Is Bone Density the Definitive Risk?

Abnormal bone density is at the top of most lists of osteoporosis risk factors, but it may not be the most important one after all. In *Food and Our Bones*, Annemarie Colbin references a study by Dr. Steven Cummings. In 1995, his group found that bone density was not the leading risk factor in a group of over-sixty-five-year-old women. Instead, the following were the predominant ways of inducing porous bones and subsequent fractures:

- Smoking
- Drugs, such as sleeping pills and tranquilizers causing dizziness and falls
- Vision problems, which cause falls
- History of overactive thyroid gland, which breaks down bone
- Above-normal height
- Need to hold arms of chair to rise indicating lack of muscle strength, which is important for bone strength
- High pulse rate, which is another indication of overactive thyroid

Without even looking at bone density levels, women having five of these seven risk factors had a 10 percent chance of breaking a hip over the next five years. With two or fewer risk factors, the chance of having a hip fracture was only 1 percent. Smoking is probably the worst risk factor because it increases other risk factors. Smokers tend to get less exercise, be in poorer health, be thinner, and have a higher pulse rate. The authors of the Cummings study made the following recommendations to help prevent osteoporosis: Maintain body weight, walk for exercise, avoid long-acting benzodiazepines (tranquilizers), minimize caffeine intake, and treat impaired visual function.[32]

The Bone Pause

The herbalist Susun Weed reported on the "bone pause" in her book *The Menopausal Years*. She tells us of the research that shows "[f]or about five years right immediately around menopause, the bones apparently reject calcium, giving rise to the belief that ERT, taken as soon as menopause begins and continued for several decades, is the only hope for women who want to avoid broken bones. But bones begin absorbing calcium once again when this 'Bone-pause' is past."

She also reminds us that ERT does not improve the creation of new bone cells; it merely slows down bone cell death. Then, when you stop ERT, the rate of bone loss can increase if you don't have other important factors in place, such as exercise and plenty of green vegetables and, according to Susun, herbs with a high mineral content.

Susun really puts osteoporosis into perspective when she notes, "Bone loss during one premenopausal month without menses is the equivalent of one year's bone-loss postmenopausally." Which means that if you are estrogen dominant and experience anovulatory cycles, you are already hastening your bone loss!

To prevent osteoporosis in perimenopause means that we must treat estrogen dominance and normalize progesterone levels, as well as encourage a bone-healthy diet and supplement program.

Homocysteine as a Risk Factor for Osteoporosis

Homocysteine is a normal amino acid produced as a byproduct of protein digestion. In elevated amounts, homocysteine causes "oxidized" cholesterol, which damages blood vessels. An increasing number of people seem to lack the ability to break down this amino acid. The enzyme that is necessary to break it down requires several B vitamins (folic acid, B_6, and B_{12}) and magnesium. When these nutrients are deficient, homocysteine builds up. A 2004 study finds that homocysteine elevation is a predictive factor for hip fracture in the elderly.[33] The researchers remark that elevated homocysteine "is easily modifiable by means of dietary intervention."

To Test or Not to Test

A dear friend of mine called me several months ago in a tearful panic. She's an artist, an intrepid world traveler, and an adventurer who has lived with aboriginals in the Australian outback and as a welcomed guest in "longhouses" in the wilds of Borneo. She was brought to her knees, however, by a bone density test. So many women like her do not understand bone density tests, and when told that their test is abnormal and that the only solution is a strong medication, they are caught in an awful bind.

Recently, a member of my organic CSA (community supported agriculture farm) angrily related her experience with bone density testing. She's small and pale but strong as a horse. Her doctor recommended that she get a bone density test, but she didn't realize it would be a spinal scan. She had to ask for a radiation shield for her thymus. She was very upset by the amount of radiation she might have received, especially when she later heard that she should have gotten an ultrasound scan of her heel as a preliminary screen for osteoporosis.

Diagnosing Osteoporosis

Doctors measure bone mineral density (BMD) to determine how much calcium is in our bones and equate that with porous bones and possible osteoporosis. I do have some concerns about this, because it does not take into consideration other necessary bone-builders such as magnesium. Without magnesium, calcium can't make bone! It's as simple as that. We'll talk more about the natural ways to fight osteoporosis later, but from the outset I want you to know that osteoporosis is not an inevitable result of menopause and aging.

Bone Density Tests

In order for an ordinary X-ray to diagnose bone loss, you have to have lost at least one-quarter of your bone weight. Special X-rays have been developed that are used mostly on the spine and hip because they are the most vulnerable to bone loss. These finely tuned X-rays are able to measure bone loss because they pass through soft tissue, which appears black on the X-ray film, and don't pass through calcified bone, which therefore appears white. If the bone starts to look gray and less distinct on X-rays, the radiologist knows your bone is getting thin.

Here is an overview of the different methods of measuring BMD. All of these tests, except ultrasound, use ionizing radiation, or X-rays, and are, therefore, contraindicated in pregnancy.

ULTRASOUND

Ultrasound can be used as an initial screening test for bone density. If these results are abnormal they can be confirmed with a DEXA scan. Sound waves are bounced off the test site, which is usually the heel. Unlike all of the other tests, ultrasound does not use potentially harmful radiation. It can't be used on the spine or hip, and it is not as accurate as DEXA to measure the effects of medications.

DUAL ENERGY X-RAY ABSORPTIOMETRY (DEXA)

DEXA uses two different X-ray beams to calculate the average amount of bone. Women often want to know how much radiation they are getting in a bone density test. The dosage of radiation is often compared to chest X-rays and said to be around 10 percent of the dose of a normal chest X-ray and therefore said to be very low. However, we must remember that X-ray radiation is accumulative and any amount can "potentially" cause damage at the cellular level. DEXA is mostly used for hip and spine testing. At its best, it can measure as little as 2 percent of bone loss per year. DEXA is the preferred method for following osteoporosis treatment.

PERIPHERAL DUAL ENERGY X-RAY ABSORPTIOMETRY (P-DEXA)

P-DEXA measures bone density in the wrist or heel. Some researchers think it is not as useful a measurement because it is used on bones that aren't as susceptible to fractures as the hip and spine. The machinery is portable and delivers about the same amount of radiation as a DEXA.

SINGLE X-RAY ABSORPTIOMETRY (SXA)

SXA emits a single X-ray beam. It is used to examine the heel bone or forearm and is a portable device.

DUAL PHOTON ABSORPTIOMETRY (DPA)

DPA utilizes a radioactive substance (gadolinium) that gravitates to bone, which is then picked up on X-ray.

QUANTITATIVE COMPUTED TOMOGRAPHY (QCT)

QCT is a type of CT scan that measures the density of a bone in the spine. Peripheral QCT, or PQCT, measures the density of bones in peripheral areas of the body, such as the wrist. It is much more expensive and results in a radiation exposure that is 20 to 200 times greater than the other techniques. It is also less accurate than DEXA, P-DEXA, or DPA and therefore rarely used.

What Will the Tests Tell Me?

Before being screened for osteoporosis, you may want to give some thought to what you will do if the results of bone mineral testing indicate that you are at risk for developing osteoporosis. Ask your doctor what your options are. An integrative medicine doctor will tell you about exercise, diet, and supplements for osteoporosis. A conventional doctor might think calcium, vitamin D, and Fosamax are your only options. You will have to decide what's best for you.

If you are like me and you try to avoid unnecessary X-rays and would not want to take medication as a first option, you might forgo the X-rays and radiation and just opt for the ultrasound screening test and adopt a natural approach. My reason for avoiding X-rays is that no matter how low the dose, they have the potential to alter DNA.

Unfortunately, when told by your doctor that your bones are thinning and your only option is estrogen and Fosamax, you may think your doctor must know all there is to know about osteoporosis and there must be no other options. Like my friend the world traveler, someone who leads a very healthy lifestyle, you might be thrown into a panic by your bone density test.

Because of what I know about menopause and aging and osteoporosis, I don't need a bone density test to make me exercise, lift weights, eat more calcium-rich foods, and take bone nutrients including lots of magnesium. However, a lifestyle approach may not be an option for some women who have had a lifelong history of osteoporosis risk factors. In that case some of the newer osteoporosis medications may come into play. Even so, diet, supplements, and exercise are still beneficial and may mean you can take less medication and therefore suffer fewer side effects.

✕ Estrogen for Osteoporosis

I have always been concerned about the promotion of synthetic estrogen as the "fix" for osteoporosis. This is partly because I know of the side effects, and partly because it encourages women to rely on a pill instead of what is really required—lifestyle, diet, and nutrients. If in the promotion of estrogen for osteoporosis, taking a pill is the main message, then that message will stick in a person's mind. Even if we have some idea that other things could be contributing to the problem or be part of the solution, we're all too eager to make it as easy as possible and grab quick solutions.

A typical opinion of many gynecologists in the late 1970s about estrogen causing endometrial cancer was this: "Cancer of the endometrium is by no means a fatal disease and osteoporosis can be."[34] I was shocked when I began reading editorials by doctors (mostly male) who were advising this particular tradeoff for women: either take estrogen and wait for endometrial cancer, or don't take it and die from complications of a hip fracture. Since I practiced naturopathic medicine as well as conventional medicine, I knew that estrogen was only about 10 percent of the solution.

I also knew that when a woman opted for HRT, she would always have in the back of her mind that any vaginal bleeding, breast lump, or even bone aches could be cancer. Women on HRT are also subjected to more frequent mammograms (and side effects of radiation) and endometrial biopsies. For someone on HRT, even a hint of suspicion on a mammogram or endometrial biopsy would often lead to surgery—most commonly, a breast biopsy or a hysterectomy.

In Chapter 2, I reported on the Women's Health Initiative study, which found that the only benefit of Premarin was a reduced risk of hip and other fractures. As I mentioned, when I read the full report I saw that the increased benefit for the bones cited was based on a total of six fewer hip fractures in one of the groups in the WHI study.

It is difficult for me to see how this small number of six cases could allow the authors to say that Premarin has a beneficial effect in preventing fractures in menopausal women.

Most doctors, however, will not read the full report and may keep prescribing Premarin based on the "headlines" or what they are told by drug manufacturers. What we should learn from the WHI study is that there is much more to our body and our bones than just estrogen.

Drugs for Osteoporosis

Even the FDA, prompted by the negative reports on estrogen by the WHI study, suggests, "While estrogen may be a good option for some women, new guidelines developed in 2003 by the FDA advise doctors to consider alternative treatments." They go on to say, "Estrogen-containing products should only be considered for women at significant risk of osteoporosis."[35] However, the FDA's idea of alternatives to estrogen consist of other drugs. In an FDA paper called "Boning Up on Osteoporosis," Paula Stern, Ph.D., a pharmacologist at Northwestern University Medical School in Chicago, is quoted as saying, "The way I visualize the ideal future is that we'll be able to give Drug X that builds up bone to where it's stronger and the risk of fracture is no longer present, then Drug Y maintains it by preventing breakdown." For a vision of my ideal future, see the osteoporosis treatment section below!

We are not suffering from a deficiency of osteoporosis drugs, but we do have a deficiency of bone nutrients and a surfeit of bad lifestyle habits that serve to create the condition. Many women are presently dealing with severe osteoporosis and may need prescription medication. But this does not mean that the drug is going to take care of everything. Eating mineral-rich foods, taking bone nutrients, and exercising will be invaluable. Remember, you can have a completely new skeleton in five years if you give it the right building blocks.

⚘ Drugs for Osteoporosis

The following drugs are being offered as the new "cure" for osteo-porosis: alendronate (Fosamax), risedronate (Actonel), raloxifene (Evista), calcitonin (Miacalcin), and teriparatide (Forteo).

Alendronate (Fosamax)

This drug was first approved in 1995 for the prevention and treatment of osteoporosis. It's a bisphosphonate, a class of drugs that destroy osteoclasts—the cells that remodel bones. Drug companies tend to label osteoclasts as cells that cause bone loss. However, that is not the whole story. Bones are constantly being remodeled. Minerals are being called out of the bones to raise blood levels where there is a need, and new minerals are laid down. Osteoclasts function to break down bone and osteoblasts create new bone. Some doctors, myself included, worry about destroying osteoclasts and interfering with proper bone remodeling just to keep extra minerals in the bones. It's easier for me to say this because I know there are alternatives to Fosamax, the ones you will learn about below.

INTENDED EFFECTS

In postmenopausal women with osteoporosis, alendronate reduces bone loss, increases bone density in both the spine and hip, and reduces the risk of spine fractures and hip fractures. Alendronate is taken as a daily or once-a-week pill.

SIDE EFFECTS

To avoid damage to the esophagus, Fosamax must be taken first thing in the morning upon awaking and at least half an hour before eating. The drug should be taken with a glass of water, and you should remain upright for half an hour after taking it. Fosamax should not be taken by people who cannot stand or sit upright or who have disorders that prevent esophageal emptying into the stomach. Fosamax can cause abdominal discomfort; muscle, bone, or joint soreness or aches; stomach upset, nausea, vomiting, diarrhea, or constipation; irritation or pain of the esophagus; stomach ulcers; eye pain; a rash; or an altered sense of taste.

Risedronate (Actonel)

This is another bisphosphonate approved for the prevention and treatment of osteoporosis.

INTENDED EFFECTS

It increases bone density, reduces the risk of spine fractures, and reduces the risk of nonspinal fractures in women with osteoporosis. Risedronate is taken as a daily or once-a-week pill.

SIDE EFFECTS

Possible side effects include abdominal discomfort; stomach upset, vomiting, nausea, or diarrhea; headache; and muscle or joint soreness or aches.

Raloxifene (Evista)

This is one of a relatively new group of drugs known as selective estrogen receptor modulators, or SERMs. These drugs are not estrogens, but they have estrogen-like effects on bone and supposedly no effect on breast tissue and uterine tissue.

INTENDED EFFECTS

Raloxifene has been shown to prevent bone loss, have beneficial effects on bone mass, and reduce the risk of spine fractures. It is taken as a tablet once a day.

SIDE EFFECTS

Side effects may include low estrogen and high estrogen effects; these include hot flashes, sweating, clot formation in some blood vessels, muscle soreness, weight gain, or a rash. This drug has not been used long enough or tested long enough to determine if it can cause breast or uterine cancer.

Calcitonin (Miacalcin)

This is a hormone involved in calcium regulation and bone metabolism. It is taken as a single daily nasal spray or as an injection under the skin. Calcitonin is only approved for treatment of osteoporosis in women who are at least five years beyond menopause.

INTENDED EFFECTS

Calcitonin slows bone loss and increases spinal bone density. Some patients report that calcitonin also relieves pain from bone fractures. The effects of calcitonin on fracture risk are still unclear.

SIDE EFFECTS

Injected calcitonin may cause an allergic reaction. Side effects may include flushing of the face and hands, increased urinaration frequency, nausea, and skin rash. Nasal calcitonin may cause a runny nose and other signs of nasal irritation.

Teriparatide (Forteo)

FDA has approved teriparatide (Forteo), the first drug for stimulating new bone formation. The drug is intended for use in postmenopausal women and in men with a high risk of bone fracture. Forteo is a synthetic form of parathyroid hormone (PTH). Human PTH is the primary regulator of calcium and phosphate metabolism in bones. The synthetic hormone is given by subcutaneous injection once daily for a period of up to twenty-four months.

INTENDED EFFECTS
After three months of therapy, Forteo increases bone mineral density and reduces fracture risk.

SIDE EFFECTS
As the drug information says, adverse events may include (but are not limited to) the following: pain, headache, asthenia, neck pain, hypertension, angina, fainting, nausea, constipation, dizziness, depression, insomnia, and vertigo. We have no way of knowing the long-term effects of Forteo since clinical trials only lasted an average of nineteen months.

Sodium Fluoride

You may have heard of a salt of fluoride, sodium fluoride, being used to treat osteoporosis. It was thought to stimulate new bone formation; however, research showed that the new bone was abnormal. It was more brittle and weaker than normal bone. Its use has been largely curtailed.

Lifelong Calcium

Since our bone mass is established in our early twenties, it is important to get sufficient calcium when we are young. As mentioned above, that may be next to impossible unless parents take back control of their children's diets. But don't feel that if you didn't have enough calcium when you were young, it's all over. There is much evidence that eating calcium-rich foods and taking the right supplements will increase your bone mass—remember, a new skeleton every five years. It is also important to remember that even though calcium is considered to be the single most important dietary factor in osteoporosis, it is not the only factor.

The RDA (recommended daily allowance) for calcium is 1,000 milligrams for perimenopause and 1,200 milligrams in menopause. Natural food experts Paul Pitchford (author of *Healing With Whole Foods*), Annemarie Colbin (*Food and Our Bones*), and Susun Weed (*The Menopausal Years*) have shown that you can get enough calcium in your diet to prevent osteoporosis and to build bone mass. The following list of high calcium foods is adapted from lists in my book *Menopause Naturally* and in *Healing with Whole Foods*.

Calcium Foods: in Milligrams

Sea Vegetables

hijiki—3.5 oz. = 1,400

wakame—3.5 oz. = 1,300

kelp—3.5 oz. = 1,099

kombu—3.5 oz. = 800

nori—3.5 oz. = 260

Dairy

brick cheese—3.5 oz. = 682

yogurt—3.5 oz. = 121

milk—3.5 oz. = 119

Vegetables, Soy, and Beans

dried wheat grass or barley grass—3.5 oz. = 514

bok choy—1 cup = 252

broccoli stalk—1 medium = 158

dandelion greens—½ cup cooked = 147

tofu—½ cup = 145

blackstrap molasses—1 tbsp = 140

turnip—1 cup cooked = 126

collards—½ cup cooked = 110

kale—½ cup cooked = 103

dried beans, cooked (white, kidney, soy, etc.)—1 cup = 95 to 110

spinach—½ cup cooked = 88

broccoli—½ cup cooked = 72

beet greens—½ cup cooked = 7

Baked Foods

soy flour—½ cup =132

corn muffin—1 medium = 96

whole wheat bread—1 slice = 50

Seafood

sardines with bones—2 oz. = 240

clams—¾ can = 62

oysters—20 medium = 300

salmon with bones—½ can (220 g) = 284

scallops—6 = 115

Nuts and Seeds

hazelnuts—3.5 oz. =209

almonds—½ cup =175

brazil nuts—½ cup = 128

sesame seeds—½ cup =76

Fruit

rhubarb, cooked—½ cup = 200

As you can see, the highest amounts of calcium are found in sea vegetables; however, it is next to impossible for anyone to eat 3.5 ounces (almost ½ cup) of sea vegetables at any one sitting! The only restaurants where you will find sea vegetables are Japanese sushi bars or health food restaurants. Sea vegetables can be found in most health food stores. They are normally cooked into soups or as a side dish with rice and vegetables.

Dairy is the next highest source of calcium. However, many people, me included, can't digest it in any form. It can cause gas and excessive mucus, which leads to a cold. Some people just don't have the necessary lactase enzymes to break down milk sugar; others may be allergic to the casein protein in milk. For women struggling with estrogen dominance, dairy may be part of the problem, not part of the solution. We also have to consider the tremendous amount of hormones and antibiotics that are regularly fed to cows, leaving measurable residues in the milk. Cows are injected with genetically engineered bovine growth hormone to increase milk production. This unnatural process creates inflammation or mastitis in the cow's udder and means even more antibiotics have to be used to prevent infection.

In order to find out if you are dairy-sensitive, eliminate it from your diet for two weeks, then eat several servings of cheese and milk in one day and see if you have a reaction. It could be an immediate reaction—nausea, vomiting, pain in the stomach—or a delayed reaction with mucus buildup in the sinuses, diarrhea, constipation, fatigue, or bowel pain.

Calcium Inhibitors

You should also know the list of foods and beverages that drain minerals from the body. The biggest drain is on calcium and magnesium. As you will see below, magnesium is just as important as calcium in building bone.

- Coffee
- Soft drinks
- Diuretics
- Excess protein, especially meat
- Refined sugar or too much of any concentrated sweetener or sweet-flavored food
- Alcohol
- Cigarettes
- Too little or too much exercise
- Excess salt
- The nightshade vegetables: tomatoes, potatoes, eggplant, and bell peppers

Magnesium Deficiency

Since researching my book *The Miracle of Magnesium*, I have become very concerned about the state of magnesium deficiency in our population. Magnesium is a required cofactor in over 350 enzymes in the body from energy production to relaxing muscles and including all things to do with bones. About 60 to 65 percent of all our magnesium is housed in our bones and teeth and it is there for a specific purpose. Susan Brown, Ph.D., Director of the Osteoporosis Education Project in Syracuse, New York, warns, "[T]he use of calcium supplementation in the face of magnesium deficiency can lead to a deposition of calcium in the soft tissue such as the joints, promoting arthritis, or in the kidney, contributing to kidney stones."[36]

Magnesium's role in bone health is multifaceted:

- Adequate levels of magnesium are essential for the absorption and metabolism of calcium.
- Magnesium stimulates a particular hormone, calcitonin, that helps to preserve bone structure and draws calcium out of the blood and soft tissues back into the bones, preventing some forms of arthritis and kidney stones.
- Magnesium suppresses another bone hormone called parathyroid, preventing it from breaking down bone.
- Magnesium converts vitamin D into its active form so that it can help calcium absorption.
- Magnesium is also required to activate an enzyme that is required to form new calcium crystals.
- Magnesium regulates active calcium transport.

Magnesium Content of Selected Foods*
in Milligrams per 3.5 oz. (100 gm., or 10-tablespoon) serving

Kelp	760	Dulse	220
Wheat bran	490	Filberts	184
Wheat germ	336	Peanuts	175
Almonds	270	Millet	162
Cashews	267	Wheat grain	160
Molasses	258	Pecan	142
Yeast, brewer's	231	English walnuts	131
Buckwheat	229	Rye	115
Brazil nuts	225	Tofu	111

*From *The Miracle of Magnesium*, Ballantine, 2003.

Herb Sources of Magnesium
in Milligrams per 3.5 oz. (100 gm)

Nettles	860	Dulse	220
Burdock root (Arctium lappa)	537	Dandelion (Taraxacum officinale)	157
Chickweed	529		

The Osteoporosis Prevention Lifestyle

Here are some rules to follow to lessen your chances of having osteoporosis:

1. Substitute herbal tea, preferably noncaffeinated, for coffee.
2. Eat small meals and chew well to avoid the need for antacids.
3. Drink pure water from a filtered source, instead of soda pop.
4. Avoid steroid drugs; find natural substitutes.
5. Don't smoke.
6. Only drink alcohol occasionally.

The Osteoporosis Prevention Diet

The best diet for osteoporosis follows from the advice of both Paul Pitchford and Annemarie Colbin. They, and many other health advocates, are concerned about the high proportion of animal protein in the Western diet. In my naturopathic training I learned that our ability to digest protein diminishes with age. There are several ways to handle this: cut back on your animal protein intake; take digestive enzymes and hydrochloric acid tablets; and increase your intake of free-range eggs and bean, pea, nut, seed, and plant sources of protein.

Before I hit menopause I used to eat everybody under the table—chicken, fish, lamb, and some free-range beef were my main protein choices. Then I found that I didn't need to eat as much. In taking care of my adrenal glands as part of my menopause program, I realized I wasn't hypoglycemic anymore and didn't need to eat four and five meals a day. In the process I found a "balanced nutrition" powder that I use morning and night. Its basic ingredient is whole eggs, and since taking that I find I don't really crave animal protein like I used to—I seem to be getting what I need from my powder. Eating less animal protein takes the pressure off my digestive enzymes.

Most nutritionists recommend the curtailment of white flour products and sweets in our diet. Not only are they devoid of nutrition, but they also drain important nutrients from the body, which have to come out in abundance in order to digest them and eliminate them because they have none of their own. As an aside—that's why raw vegetables are so valued, they contain their own enzymes and nutrients and help in their own digestion. Try this experiment: put a raw carrot on a plate and it rots naturally, put a fast food hamburger, bun and all, on a plate and with all the preservatives and additives, it can last for months. Colbin and Pitchford also suggest we avoid overeating the nightshade vegetables (potatoes, tomatoes, eggplant, peppers) and consume a greater variety of vegetables and high-quality fats. I'll outline this diet in Chapter 11.

Osteoporosis Prevention Supplements

The following list of nutrients with recommended dosages are for your information only. They are not given as a treatment protocol. If you begin an osteoporosis supplement program, be sure to do so in conjunction with a health care provider. The list may look long, but it is not inclusive; each nutrient listed has a range of other nutrients that it requires for proper utilization. The end result is that all nutrients in the body are necessary for proper maintenance of bone.

Boron—10 mg per day. Boron promotes proper calcium metabolism and prevents urinary calcium loss. It also increases levels of natural estradiol in the blood, which helps promote bone health. The best sources of boron are organic fruits, vegetables, and nuts.

Calcium—1,000 to 1,500 mg. Try to obtain half your calcium from calcium-rich foods and half from supplements of calcium citrate. Leave calcium carbonate—including Tums—in the rocks from which it comes. It doesn't dissolve and immediately neutralizes stomach acid, which you need for absorbing calcium in the first place—as well as for absorbing your food. Calcium carbonate also causes constipation, kidney stones, and soft tissue and joint buildup of calcium, leading to arthritis and muscle pain.

Copper—3 mg per day.

Magnesium—800 to 1,000 mg. The recommended dosage for magnesium is only about half of what we really need. If you aren't eating magnesium-rich foods you must take supplements—even then you may only get half of what you need. Magnesium in high amounts is a laxative: magnesium oxide is for people with constipation, magnesium citrate is the most widely used, and magnesium glycinate is for people who have loose bowel movements.

Manganese—10 mg per day.

Microcrystalline Hydroxyapatite (MCHC) is a calcium supplement that may prevent and repair bone loss. MCHC is a whole bone extract, or food, that provides calcium in a bioavailable form. It is different from bone meal. Bone meal is to be avoided since it may contain lead.

Vitamin D—800 IU per day. Vitamin D is a prohormone, which is necessary for the absorption of calcium. Twenty minutes of sunshine a day, without sunscreen, provides a daily dose of vitamin D.

Vitamin C—1,000 mg in a complex of bioflavins.

Vitamin A—10,000 IU per day.

Vitamin B_6—50 mg per day.

Vitamin K—1,000 micrograms per day. Vitamin K is crucial to calcium absorption. Yogurt, molasses, leafy greens, green tea, kelp, and nettles are important food sources.

Vitamin B_{12}—500 micrograms per day.

Zinc—15 mg per day. Taking higher doses of zinc over long periods of time can result in low levels of copper.

Osteoporosis Prevention Exercise

A few decades ago, before there was much research on exercise and osteoporosis, it was thought that heavy physical exercise was the only way to build bone. I learned an important lesson around 1984 when a patient of mine was told she had very thin bones that were on the verge of breaking. She didn't want to take estrogen or any other drug or supplement. She had been told by a martial arts teacher that the standing postures of chi kung would increase bone mass. She also went on a diet of calcium-rich foods. Everyone was amazed when, after three months, her bone mass had improved. At the time her improvement seemed like a miracle, but then we learned that most exercise—even isotonic exercise where you hold a posture for a minute at a time, as in chi kung—can activate bone metabolism and lay down extra calcium and other minerals.

The following list of exercises should give you some ideas for your own program.

- Walking, at a good pace.
- Jogging: The best surface to jog on is a mini-trampoline.

- Yoga
- Tai chi
- Chi kung
- Biking
- Swimming
- Pilates
- T-Tapp: See Chapter 11 for a discussion about this exercise.

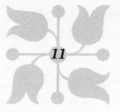

11

The Hormonal Diet and Exercise Plan

WHAT I'VE ALLUDED TO throughout this book is a diet and exercise plan to support your liver, adrenals, thyroid, heart, and bones. It's a tall order but one that needs to be fulfilled. In the process, you need to kick out the chemicals and unleash your energy with a side benefit of losing weight.

✤ Every Woman's Diet

You may have already begun to change your diet and detoxify after reading Chapter 7, and you may have decided to eliminate Candida after identifying yourself in the Candidiasis picture described in Chapter 8. If so, you may be experiencing less gas and bloating, and may even have lost some weight. You may have noticed less mucus and clearer sinuses. This is only the beginning of feeling better, a feeling that will extend to all systems of your body as you become less toxic and less overloaded with processed foods. The natural human tendency of "wanting more" can now be geared toward wanting more energy, more body tone, more confidence in your own ability to create a healthier you.

The Standard American Diet (SAD)

Keep this in mind: "In 1970 Americans spent about $6 billion on fast food; in 2000 they spent more than $110 billion dollars. Americans now spend more money on fast food than on higher education, personal computers, computer software, or new cars. They spend more on fast food than on movies, books, magazines, newspapers, videos, and recorded music—combined." Eric Schlosser, who wrote that in his book *Fast Food Nation*, is mightily concerned about the amount of processed, junk food we eat. Remember this quote next time you wonder to yourself, "Why does everyone seem so sick!"

I've been promising a diet for menopause throughout the book; however, the optimal diet won't just be about hormonal balance. This diet will help you lose weight, decrease your risk of heart disease, cancer, and diabetes—and along with the calcium- and magnesium-rich foods in Chapter 10, it will help prevent osteoporosis and arthritis. I don't mean to suggest that the same diet is going to suit everyone; it's going to take some experimentation on your part to see whether you gravitate toward more of the protein food group or the carbohydrate food group. What will become clear is that we all have to avoid the refined carbohydrates—those are the foods that are causing much of the problems with obesity, insulin resistance, and even estrogen dominance.

OK, let's dive in. Good health begins with water.

Water

When I was recently asked to give a presentation at a spa retreat for businesswomen, I was very excited. Here was a collection of women who were making a difference in the world. It comes as no surprise that women are in charge of 95 percent of the health care decisions and food purchases in the family. Knowing this, I wanted to tell them how they and their families could lead healthier lives by making the right choices in diet and health care. It came as quite a shock when the predominant response to my seminar was, "I learned a lot, but of all the options for taking care of my health, all I can manage to do with all my time constraints is drink more water."

No home-cooked meals, no organic food, no supplements, no time for exercise, no time for meditation—all I can do is drink more water! I was the one who got an education at that spa. I realized that women are so stressed having to take care of both business and family that they don't have time to take care of themselves. Even worse, they are partly responsible for promoting the fast-food lifestyle!

Women don't have time to cook so, by default, it's up to fast-food restaurants to feed us inferior food. We allow our kids to drink soda and to eat ice cream and junk food—much like the pacifiers that we give babies. As another pacifier, we also allow too much mind-numbing TV. Junk food and junk entertainment that advertises junk food are incredibly inferior substitutes for a decent diet and family interaction.

But back to water—I reconciled that if I got the message across about water than I had, at least, done something. After all:

- 75 percent of all people are chronically dehydrated.
- In 37 percent of us, the thirst mechanism is so weak that it is often mistaken for hunger.
- Even MILD dehydration will slow down one's metabolism by as much as 3 percent.
- According to one university study, one glass of water shuts down midnight hunger pangs for almost 100 percent of the dieters studied.
- Lack of water is the number one trigger of daytime fatigue.

- Preliminary research indicates that eight to ten glasses of water a day could significantly ease back and joint pain for up to 80 percent of sufferers.
- A mere 2 percent drop in body water can trigger fuzzy short-term memory, trouble with basic math, and difficulty focusing on a computer screen.
- Drinking five glasses of water daily decreases the risk of colon cancer by 45 percent, plus it can slash the risk of breast cancer by 79 percent, and one is 50 percent less likely to develop bladder cancer.

The best formula that I've heard for how much water we need to consume is this: one half your weight in ounces of water. I'm about 100 pounds, so I need 50 ounces a day.

OK, time for a water break! I'm always asked about what type of water to use. With the amount of chlorine and fluoride in modern water supplies it seems prudent to invest in a water purifier. I recommend this above bottled water—because ultimately we don't know the source or the quality of the latter. A good water purifier should guarantee elimination of chemicals, asbestos, heavy metals, and microorganisms. I use a purifier that filters to the level of ½ micron, and that removes chlorine, fluoride, asbestos, and heavy metals.

❧ Diet

An osteoporosis-prevention diet is outlined in Chapter 10, but in order to prevent the disease you have to start young. If our bones are formed by age twenty, that means our children have to eat calcium- and magnesium-rich foods. Unfortunately it seems that the last thing that most young people want to do is eat well!

I started a CSA (community supported agriculture group) where I live. Members buy a share in an organic farm and every week for six months, from June to November, the farmers deliver crates of delicious vegetables and fruits. Parents join because they love the food, but many of them don't rejoin the next year because they say their kids just won't eat the vegetables. Their brains and appetites have been hijacked by junk food!

Personally, I do not think food should be negotiable. You are what you eat and your brain is also what you eat. There are several ways you can educate your children and grandchildren about diet. Perhaps the movie *Super Size Me* will appeal to them. That "docudrama" shows the weight gain, abnormal blood fat levels, and abnormal liver blood tests in one person on a thirty-day McDonald's diet. Episodes of throwing up after a Big Mac, dizziness, lack of energy, and irritability aptly demonstrate what such a defective diet can do to a person.

Diet Experiments

Whenever I get a chance, I offer kids their own personal experiment. With their parents' permission, I ask children to go on a six-day junk-free diet—no sugar, no soda, no chips, no candy, no cake, no donuts. Then on Saturday, they are allowed to have all the candy, soda, and snacks they want. Being off junk food for most of the week clears most of their systems, and the overload of sugar on Saturday makes most of them sick all day Sunday. Finally, they can clearly see and feel exactly what this food is doing to their bodies. Most of them swear off junk food after that experiment.

Another way to get kids to understand what they are eating is the mummification experiment. Buy a cheeseburger and fries at any of the junk food establishments—most people choose McDonald's. Place the burger and fries on a shelf and leave them there. What you learn is that these foods are so artificial that they will never rot. They will sit there looking the same as on the day they were bought for months at a time. Most people, young or old, get the message that this is not the way food should be. Such junk food has no living enzymes in it to help break it down in the body. The strain on our digestion begins immediately with food that is dead. It taxes our stomach acids and our pancreatic enzymes, and it clogs up our bowels; the sugar throws off our insulin, and the fat clogs up our heart. The chemical preservatives, binders, fillers, colorants, and taste enhancers put a severe strain on the liver's detoxification systems. That's why after thirty days liver blood tests show liver damage.

Mice on McDonald's

I've heard that the following experiment has been banned by some school systems because it is cruel and unusual punishment to animals. Feed one mouse junk food and another a wholesome diet. Within weeks the junk-food mouse looks frazzled, bedraggled, and sick, while the wholesome mouse looks perfectly healthy.

I also ask young people if they would feed their dog ice cream, cookies, cakes, soda, or pizza. The answer is always a resounding "No way." The next obvious question I ask is "So, why do you think it's OK for you to eat it?" I then tell them about an experiment from the 1970s in which researchers from the University of Alabama under the guidance of Emmanuel Cheraskin, a noted medical doctor and dentist, fed one group of rats sugar-coated cereal and another group the cardboard cereal box. You guessed it. The rats that ate the box were healthier than the rats that ate the cereal. When you eat junk food, not only do you eat foods that are detrimental to your health but you take valuable stomach room away from good foods.

Diet Before Supplements

The supplement industry is built around the fact that people eat poorly. But even if you eat an excellent organic diet, you still need supplements to deal with stress and environment toxins. I certainly take my share. However, supplements are not the place to start.

When you eat a good diet you are getting the effect of hundreds of nutrient components instead of one single nutrient.

Why White Flour and Sugar Are Not Your Friends

Sure, when they're all dressed up as cakes and pastries, white flour and sugar put on a good show. They're equated with love and romance; they can even give you a buzz and make you feel high. But refined flour products and sugar can make you crash, too. It's called hypoglycemia, or low blood sugar, and it's something you really want to avoid—it's the first step on the way to diabetes.

A nutrition educator I know tells her clients "It costs nothing to give up sugar." It's the first step to recovering your health. Sugar underlies the recent upsurge in the insulin-resistance diseases. The spiking of blood sugar when you drink a soda triggers a release of insulin from the pancreas. At any one time there is only about one teaspoon's worth of sugar in our bloodstream.

The dramatic rise in blood sugar—from the normal one teaspoon—to ten teaspoons causes hypersecretion of insulin. If you drink sodas and eat sugary products on a daily basis, it's only a matter of time before insulin and glucose are constantly elevated. Rapidly rising and falling blood sugar creates a negative feedback cycle, where high levels of sugar in the blood stimulate the release of adrenaline.

Adrenaline stimulates cortisol release, and cortisol causes a craving for calories. Even if you have just finished eating, cortisol will make you feel famished. I mentioned earlier that it is impossible for someone to lose weight if they are under constant stress because cortisol keeps demanding to be fed.

Feeding Fat

High insulin levels also shut down the ability of the body to burn fat. This occurs because insulin is elevated when sugar and simple carbohydrates like donuts are eaten—simply having an elevated sugar means the body doesn't need to burn fat for energy. It has enough energy from the carbs, so why go to all the trouble to burn fat? That's why the no-carb diets work initially; the body first uses up all your carbohydrate stores, which also happens to release a lot of water. Then fat burning begins as more energy is required to keep the body working. The trouble is, with no or very low carbs you can start breaking down muscle as well, and that's not a good thing.

Syndrome X

High insulin levels are responsible for a dizzying array of chronic diseases. One symptom complex called Syndrome X is characterized by obesity, elevated triglycerides, high cholesterol, hypertension, and Type 2 diabetes. Even children, after consuming candy and soda for a decade, are developing adult-onset Type 2 diabetes and have *Acanthosis nigricans* skin markings. I found out about acanthosis while researching a condition called polycystic ovarian syndrome (PCOS). People with PCOS have brown-black marks on their neck, elbows, knees, and knuckles due to high insulin levels—and so do our obese children.

Hypoglycemia

I've mentioned that people under adrenal stress are at high risk for hypoglycemia. However, it seems to be even more common in menopausal women. Carbohydrate metabolism is affected by the decreased progesterone secretion in the second half of the menstrual cycle in perimenopausal women, especially if there is an anovulatory cycle that produces little progesterone. This leads to changes in the tolerance to sugar, which means that you get hungry when your blood sugar is still high. Essentially, you crave more sugar and carbohydrates; partly it's because cortisol is elevated and causes sugar cravings. Perhaps it's also part of the adaptation to menopause where we need to gain ten pounds to help make our postmenopausal hormones. It's gotten out of control, however, in our culture, because carbs are everywhere and we can't seem to resist them.

Saying No to Sugar

Resist them you must. It is the high sugar levels leading to insulin resistance that is at the basis of our epidemic of obesity, diabetes, hypertension, heart disease, and stroke. Even cancer thrives on sugar, and the first treatment of any cancer should be "no more sugar." If you give in to your cravings for carbohydrates with the usual denial tactics—"I deserve this, I work so hard" or "It's only one slice" or "I need sugar to keep up my strength"—then you are only fooling your brain, and not your body.

I pulled my usual excuse out of the hat just the other day. When my husband and I "blow" our normally very healthy diet, we call it an "experiment." My experiment was to buy a 3.5 ounce chocolate bar—and eat the whole thing. Even more denial went into this experiment because I bought dark chocolate, 73 percent cacao, and it was organic. So what could be the harm? I ate it driving home from the health food store and we went for a long walk before it hit me. I could barely finish the walk. I felt shaky and weak and headachy because the sugar high changed into a sugar low and I had an attack of hypoglycemia. The high amount of sugar triggered an excess of insulin that pulled too much sugar out of my blood into the cells, leaving me shaky from low blood sugar. Fortunately, I knew what was occurring, but most people don't and can get caught up in the medical system when they try to explain symptoms of hypoglycemia to their doctors.

✂ Hypoglycemia and Menopause

The following chart compares symptoms of hypoglycemia and menopause. They are remarkably similar. The chart also gives you an indication that keeping your blood sugar under control can help alleviate some of the symptoms of menopause, because hypoglycemia symptoms on top of menopause symptoms will just make the latter seem so much worse.

Hypoglycemia	*Menopause*
Fatigue	Fatigue
Changes in energy level	Changes in energy level
Faintness	
Falling asleep after meals	
Less mentally alert	
Memory failure	Memory lapses
Rapid heartbeat	Racing heart
Mood changes	Mood changes
Irritability	Bursts of anger
Nervousness	Panic attacks
Anxieties	Anxieties
Depression	Depression
Shakiness	
Tremors	
Hunger pangs	
Sugar cravings	Sugar cravings
Giddiness	Head feels fuzzy
Lightheaded, dizzy	Lightheaded, dizzy
Headaches	Headaches
Hot flashes	Hot flashes

Hypoglycemia	Menopause (continued)
Fatigue	Fatigue
Joint pain	Joint pain
Backache	Backache
Muscle pain	Muscle pain
Chronic indigestion	Indigestion
Obesity	Weight gain
Blurred vision	Blurred vision
Allergies	Allergies
Noise and light sensitivity	Noise and light sensitivity
Itching and crawling sensations on skin	Itching and crawling sensations on skin
Gasping for breath	Gasping for breath
Lack of sex drive	Lack of sex drive

Insulin Reacts to Sugar

As mentioned in Chapter 5, hypoglycemia, or low blood sugar, is an insulin reaction to an elevated blood sugar. Your blood sugar becomes quickly elevated if you eat a donut and coffee; drink a soda (ten teaspoons of sugar); simply have white toast slathered with jam; or eat a 3.5 ounce chocolate bar! Insulin floods out of the pancreas to deal with the high levels and tries its best to corral all the sugar into our cells—with the excess going into fat storage. When the blood sugar goes through a rapid increase and then a precipitous decline, adrenaline is stimulated to make sure the blood sugar does not fall too low, leading to unconsciousness.

Fight or Flight

Adrenaline is mainly trying to release sugar that is stored as glycogen in the liver and muscles. However, at the same time, it triggers a fight-or-flight reaction. This is where the scary stuff begins. Adrenaline pumping into your blood, seemingly for no reason, gives you all the signs and symptoms of being frightened, which you interpret as an anxiety attack. Many phobias and fears are born from a solitary low blood sugar attack. Most psychiatrists don't ask what you were eating when you had your attack; they just dig for the psychological causes.

Glucose Tolerance Test

Medically, hypoglycemia is only recognized if the blood sugar drops below a certain range. Normal blood sugar is about 100 milligrams per deciliter (one tenth of a liter, mg/dL); hypoglycemia is defined at 50 milligrams per deciliter (mg/dL) or lower and is usually found on a glucose tolerance test (GTT). It is very important to diagnose this condition properly. There is much controversy over how to do a proper GTT. I have found the best results with the following protocol.

- Do the test in the morning after a 12- to 14-hour fast (water is acceptable).
- Take the initial glucose and insulin blood levels.
- Eat a high-carbohydrate meal (one banana, one orange, several dates and figs) instead of the straight sugar drink.
- Keep a journal of symptoms throughout the test.
- Take a half-hour glucose and insulin level and repeat every hour for five hours.

A continuous measurement of blood sugar and insulin would give the most accurate picture because regular testing intervals can miss the peak of blood sugar from the sugar meal and the precipitous drop. The standard 2-hour GTT, designed to diagnose diabetes and insulin resistance, usually misses hypoglycemia. Many doctors don't understand the hypoglycemia picture. In medical school I was told it was a very rare condition that occurred when people had tumors that secreted excessive amounts of insulin. We were not prepared for the onslaught of such a highly processed and sugared diet that created "reactive" hypoglycemia—reactive means that the blood sugar is reacting to a high sugar meal.

Treating Hypoglycemia

The treatment of hypoglycemia is not a sugary drink or candy, as many doctors have suggested. It's a matter of keeping the blood sugar stabilized by *not* eating sugar and refined white flour products. You don't want high sugar levels triggering insulin and causing precipitous plunges. Cycling of highs and lows of blood sugar causes significant strain on both the pancreas and adrenal glands. If you continue to eat sugary foods, day after day, your cells will put up the "no admittance" sign to insulin. Insulin and sugar levels will keep rising and cause damage to eyes, heart, and kidneys, and the adrenal glands become overworked dealing with low blood sugar episodes.

Small frequent meals of complex carbohydrates and protein is the appropriate diet to pursue. In someone with severe hypoglycemia, fruit is limited to two pieces a day of high fiber apples and pears. Complex carbohydrates include vegetables, whole grains, lentils, beans, peas, nuts, and seeds. Protein includes fish, chicken, and fermented soy products (tempeh, miso).

Supplements that are helpful in treating hypoglycemia include:

- B vitamin complex to support the nervous system: 50 milligrams, one to two a day in a nonyeast base
- A good multivitamin and mineral
- Pantothenic acid, a B vitamin that supports the adrenal glands: 500 milligrams, one to three a day, especially important for people whose adrenal glands are exhausted
- An herbal formula for adrenal support
- Chromium, a mineral that has been shown to assist glucose tolerance and balance: 200 micrograms per day

Sugar Substitutes Are Not the Answer

If you're thinking, OK, fine, I won't eat sugar, I'll use sugar sub-stitutes—that would be a mistake. The most widely used artificial sweetener, aspartame (Equal, Spoonful, NutraSweet), is made partly from methanol, also called wood alcohol, which causes blindness. If that isn't bad enough, when aspartame reaches body temperature, it breaks down into formaldehyde. It's just not safe and is responsible for over ninety-two adverse side effects, including headaches, brain tumors, skin itching, rashes, infertility, diabetes, mood swings, and, ironically, weight gain!

All the other sugar substitutes are also synthesized chemicals and have their own list of problems. The one acceptable natural sweetener is Stevia. All artificial sweeteners—no matter the adver-tising hype—are synthetic and put strain on the body. Stevia is pro-duced from the leaves of a plant that grows in South America and is 200 times sweeter than sugar. It's very safe and has been used commercially in Japan for decades. For no apparent reason the FDA won't allow it to be labeled as a sugar substitute, but it is available as a supplement in health stores. Try the drops or the powder and see what's best for sweetening your tea or baking. Once you balance your body with the right diet and nutrients, however, you will be surprised to find that you no longer have those sugar or carbohy-drate cravings.

Fat and Sugar Labeling

I've talked about the many ways our bodies cling to fat. One factor is the buildup of chemicals in our fat storage sites so that any time you try to lose weight, you create a chemical factory in your blood, making you feel yucky. Another factor is the natural tendency for the body to store fat to help make more estrogen. The most com-mon estrogen in postmenopause is estrone, which is created in fatty tissue. A factor we shouldn't forget is the shameless marketing of billions of dollars worth of fat-filled or sugar-filled processed food.

Start reading labels. If you haven't noticed yet, a product that is sugar-free is high in fat; a product that is labeled fat-free is twice as high in sugar. They've got us by our taste buds! Another labeling trick is that sugar and simple carbohydrates are listed in grams. But most people in the United States don't know that there are four grams in one teaspoon. By knowing this simple fact you can read a soft drink label and see forty grams of carbs and realize that means ten teaspoons of sugar! You might think that yogurt is a healthy snack—until you read the label saying that there are 28 grams or seven teaspoons of sugar in a small 3-ounce serving. You'll also be surprised to read ketchup labels with sugar as the first ingredient. Labels by law have to list ingredients in order of weight. So, a labeling trick of manufacturers is to use three different types of sugar in a product and label them as three separate entities. If they were all added up, sugar would be the top ingredient, but as three separate sugars they are hidden within the other ingredients.

Dieting Affects the Thyroid

The first rule: Don't starve yourself. Starvation translates into calorie restriction. Such behavior can change the way the thyroid is converted from its more inactive state (T3) to its more active state (T4). Unfortunately, anyone who has been dieting for years has made their body adapt to times of food deprivation. For example, most people can go without breakfast and maybe lunch but then must eat something around dinnertime. Skipping meals teaches the body how to conserve fat. If you starve all day and then at night eat a big meal and think you'll lose weight, you are in for a surprise. The food that you don't burn off before you go to sleep waltzes right into your fat cells.

This conversion is done very nicely by a specific enzyme that increases as soon as you begin to starve yourself. That's why sometimes you think you're eating "nothing" and you still gain weight. The "nothing" you're eating is being stored in your fat cells.

The stress of skipping meals translates into hormonal release of the stress hormone, cortisol. Perceiving that the body is under massive stress and needs fuel, cortisol directs the body to break down muscle protein for energy. The end result is increase in fat cells and breakdown of muscle—leaving you overweight and weak.

Eating one big meal a day, which is the usual way people diet, also affects the production of two pancreatic hormones, insulin and glucagon. Glucagon stimulates an increase in blood concentration of glucose. Because the brain depends on glucose for fuel, during times of starvation, when blood sugar levels drop, glucagon triggers the liver to release glucose stores. Erratic eating patterns lead to erratic insulin and glucagon behavior. A burst of insulin, issued to deal with a high sugar load or a large meal, can lead to elevated triglyceride levels. A drop in glucagon can paralyze the body's ability to release fat. All these imbalances lead to rapid accumulation of fat.

✤ The Menopause Lifestyle Plan

I've been promising to show you the optimum diet for hormone balance through the whole book. Finally, the time has come to unveil the menopause menu for health. It's not as "simple" as low carb or high protein. In fact, the best balanced diet is a combination of carbs and protein and fats—just like nature intended. Let's look at the various steps I've been building.

1. Detoxify your body—eliminate coffee, alcohol, and cigarettes.
2. Eliminate stress foods: sugar, white flour, and, for some, dairy.

3. Eat a healthy diet.
4. Exercise regularly.
5. Maintain a healthy outlook on life.

Detoxify

After you eliminate coffee, alcohol, and cigarettes, you may experience an aggravation of symptoms when you try to go back to old habits. In other words, once you feel better, if toxic substances are ingested you may have an unpleasant reaction to them. This immediate feedback should warn you to avoid them. This is in fact a good sign; it's the way the body encourages you to avoid the bad guys.

Remember the list from Chapter 7:

1. Identify the toxins.
2. Decrease your exposure to toxins.
3. Maximize excretion of toxins.
4. Provide nutritional support for specific detoxification pathways.
5. Reestablish intestinal flora balance.

My Personal Program

Many women talk about the extra ten pounds that they can't seem to lose. So far, I seem to have beaten that problem. I attribute it to a Body Rejuvenation Cleanse with HaloWorks Herbal Tinctures that is designed to cleanse the body of accumulated toxins and infections. I co-developed this program with Delia Quigley, a certified chef and yoga instructor.

I find also that as I get older I don't need to eat as much. I have a protein drink in the morning, a Crock-Pot grain cereal with flaxseed oil around lunch, and a big salad at dinner along with an egg dish, or pasta and shrimp, or occasionally, chicken. I make my own meals and keep most of my diet organic to avoid chemicals.

The Transition Diet

It's not enough to just give someone a list of foods to avoid and expect them to change their diet. It's much better to build a bridge between the standard American diet (SAD) with the Body Rejuvenation Cleanse—this bridge is a "transition diet." This diet is optimum for most people and far healthier than the SAD. It is derived from the Body Rejuvenation Cleanse Program.

Figure 11.1

Transition Diet

Present Diet	Transition Diet
Meat, cold cuts, hot dogs, chicken, fried fish, pork	Fish, shellfish, organic chicken, beans, tofu, tempeh, veggie burger, miso
Sugar, molasses, chocolate, candy, refined sugar desserts	Maple syrup, raw honey, Stevia, rice syrup, carob, dates, raisins
Milk, cheese, cream, coffee creamer	Rice milk, nut milk, yogurt, butter, nut butters, fermented soy yogurt, nuts, seeds
Tropical/subtropical fruits, artificial juices, sweetened teas	Organic seasonal fruits and fresh juices, unsulphured dried fruits
Coffee, black tea, soft drinks, diet drinks, alcohol, beer, wine	Organic herbal teas, green tea, mineral, spring, unfiltered water, grain coffee
Hydrogenated oils, palm oil, light olive oil, lard, GMO corn oil, canola oil, generic vegetable oil	Organic butter, coconut oil, sesame oil, flax oil, extra virgin olive oil, ghee
Refined white flour, bread, crackers, bagels, tortillas, pizza, cookies, cakes, muffins, pasta, pretzels, Danish	Wheat-free whole grain and sprouted breads, unleavened flour products, wheat-free pasta, brown rice
GMO corn chips, potato chips, other fried chips	Baked blue corn chips, air-popped popcorn, rice cakes, roasted nuts and seeds

The Transition Diet accomplishes several things—it gives you more fiber (which helps drag excess estrogen from the body); provides more nutrients; uses high quality fats and oils (that help build a healthy fatty layer that surrounds all the cells of your body including your nerve cells); and reduces intake of refined food. Let's break the diet down into the three major food groups. A balanced diet means you eat something from each group at each meal: protein, carbohydrates, and fat.

Protein

Fish, chicken, turkey, meat, legumes, beans, peas. Have only one serving a day of animal protein and two servings a day of vegetarian protein. Do your best to buy free-range, nonantibiotic, nonhormone animal protein and organic legumes, beans, and peas. Protein sustains blood sugar for two to three hours.

Carbohydrates

There are two types of carbs. Simple carbs are the refined products that can play havoc with your blood sugar. They include white flour and white sugar products: bagels, bread, cakes, cookies, etc.— all the things we think are good, but that aren't our friends! Complex carbs include grains, vegetables, beans, peas, lentils. Complex carbs are the best kind of carbs, and if you can make them organic, that's even better. Carbs are for quick energy, lasting one to two hours. Sugar can only sustain the blood sugar for one half hour.

Good sources of carbs include:

- **Whole grains:** rice, millet, rye, wheat, barley, kasha, quinoa, spelt, kamut. Choose nonwheat pasta for a change.
- **Vegetables:** broccoli, cabbage, potatoes, yams, lettuce, arugula, spinach, collards, chard, squash, onions, garlic.
- **Fruit:** pears, apples, citrus, melons, berries.

Fats and Oils

Healthy sources of fat include nuts, especially almonds, walnuts, pecans, hazelnuts; seeds, sunflower and pumpkin; avocados; butter from free-range cows; flaxseed oil on cooked cereal or salads; olive oil on salads; and coconut oil for cooking.

Fats sustain blood sugar for three to four hours. That's why you feel more full after a fatty meal. Fat became the "bad guy" when researchers began to uncover the connection between saturated fats and heart disease. Unfortunately, butter was snagged up in the ban on fats, which led to the huge commercialization of synthetic spreads such as—that's right—margarine.

I remember when I was a kid begging for the privilege of beating the little packet of red dye into the unappetizing white margarine to make a slightly more appetizing yellow spread. It took a few decades for the news to appear that the trans fatty acids made by forcing liquid vegetable oils into solid margarine were a bigger threat to health than butter ever was.

Another aspect of fat that is very important is its ability to assist the absorption of carotenoids or vitamin A. Without fat the vitamin A in salads is much less available. Adding avocado, sunflower seeds, and an oil-and-vinegar dressing greatly assists the absorption. You may think you are getting plenty of vitamin A because your salad contains carrots and broccoli, along with lettuce, but if you use a fat-free salad dressing the absorption of vitamin A from vitamin A–rich vegetables is greatly diminished.

Phytoestrogen Power Foods

Most people have a difficult time comprehending phytoestrogens. Because doctors don't understand them, many tell their breast cancer patients to avoid anything to do with estrogen—including phytoestrogen. However, phytoestrogens may be important cancer fighters and they are certainly important for balancing female hormones. *Phyto-* stands for plant, and phytoestrogens are found in over 300 different foods—so, in fact, you are eating phytoestrogens every day.

Although they can have some of the same actions as estrogens, almost none of them have the exact same structure as the estrogens we produce in our body. According to Dr. Deborah Moskowitz, writing for power-surge.com, there are a few foods that contain "steroidal estrogens (estradiol, estrone, or estriol) in small amounts: French bean, pomegranate seed, apple seed, date palm, licorice, and rice." The phytoestrogens we hear about most are isoflavones, lignans, and coumestrol. Flaxseeds, raw pumpkin seeds, red clover sprouts, and mung bean sprouts are the best ways to get these nutrients—we'll talk about soybeans separately below.

Phytoestrogens compete with estrogen for binding sites. When estrogen levels are low, phytoextrogens can act as replacement therapy. When estrogen levels are high, they bind to estrogen receptor sites that block excess estrogen and prevent estrogen dominance. We know that isoflavones, in particular, act like weak estrogens (the beneficial one—estriol) and are just strong enough to bind to breast cell receptors, blocking strong estrogens (the more harmful one—estradiol). But they aren't strong enough themselves to turn on cellular activity.

Isoflavones are extracted from soy and used in supplements for hormone health but there is a heated debate about their safety. Soy is a high-protein bean that has gotten considerable press in the last decade. With regard to menopause, some researchers believe that Japanese women do not suffer the same menopause symptoms as women in America because they benefit from the natural estrogen properties of soy. Since the uncovering of this "anecdotal" evidence, soy has been widely promoted as the "cure" for menopause in a variety of commercial products: soy milk, soy cheese, soy protein powder, and soy meat substitutes. Women are advised, mostly by soy manufacturers, to have a serving of soy every day.

However, unfermented soy is very difficult to digest. Nutritionists report that women on a high soy diet have trouble with gas and bloating. Evidence of the blocking effect of soy on thyroid hormones and the chelating effect on minerals makes some doctors uneasy about recommending so much soy. In Asian countries small amounts of fermented soy are eaten and have been eaten from childhood. This soy has gone through a long fermentation process that makes it more digestible and removes the substances that affect the thyroid and minerals. I'm one of those people who can't digest soy, so I researched this problem many years ago. I've always cautioned against the use of unfermented soy. Fermented soy products include tempeh and miso.

Diet Tips

- Eat when you're hungry.
- Eat in moderation.
- If you chew, chew, chew twenty to forty times per bite you will never have digestive problems.
- Eat your larger meals at breakfast and lunch, not at night.
- Don't drink liquids with your meals, as you will dilute your digestive enzymes and stomach acids.
- Only eat until you're 80 percent full. Give some room for the enzymes and stomach acids to do their work.

Gauging Fullness

If you don't have a sense of what being 80 percent full feels like, here are two different ways of gauging how much to eat at a meal. Animal studies show that underfeeding and caloric restriction actually lead to longevity.

USE YOUR HANDS

Have six servings of carbs, six servings of protein, and six servings of fat per day. Some say that the size of our stomach is equal to our two cupped hands held side-by-side.

- One serving of carbs is the amount of food you can fit into one hand.
- One serving of protein is the amount of food that can fit into one palm.
- One serving of fat is the size of one thumb.

USE YOUR WEIGHT

Determine your ideal weight in pounds and make that equal to the amount of carb grams you can have a day. (Here's a quick way to calculate ideal weight. Females: for 5 feet you are allowed 100 pounds, and add five pounds for every additional inch. Males: for 5 feet allow 110 pounds and add five pounds for every additional inch.)

- Half of your body weight equals the amount of protein grams you can have each day.
- Half of your protein grams equals the amount of fat grams you can have each day.

For example, if you are a 5-foot 6-inch female with small bones, a good weight is between 120 and 130 pounds. So the amount of carbs per day is 120 to 130 grams.

The amount of protein per day will then be 60 to 65 grams.

The amount of fat per day will be 30 grams.

This gives you a ratio of 50/25/25.

It's the combination and balance that's important.

✣ Menopause Menus

Morning Breakfast

2 soft-boiled eggs

1 slice rye, spelt, or kamut toast

1 piece of fruit

water or herb tea

or

turkey or chicken sausages

toasted rice mochi

1 piece of fruit

water or herb tea

or

Crock-Pot cooked cereal with berries and flax meal

water or herb tea

or

a Green Drink or Balanced Nutrition Protein Powder

Morning Snack

A Green Drink or Balanced Nutrition Powder

or

Balanced Nutrition Bar

Lunch

grilled chicken or fish

steamed vegetables or mesclun salad

with oil, vinegar, garlic, mustard dressing

brown rice

fruit

water or herb tea

✳ Menopause Menus *(continued)*

Afternoon Snack

baked corn chips

---

plain yogurt

Dinner

tuna, chicken, or egg salad on whole-wheat pita

or

1 slice of spelt bread

---

mesclun salad

---

with oil, vinegar, garlic mustard dressing

---

fruit

---

water or herb tea

or

soup

---

mesclun salad

---

oil, vinegar, garlic mustard dressing

---

fruit

---

water or herb tea

or

steamed vegetables

---

brown rice

---

fruit

---

water or herb tea

Evening Snack

---

popcorn, mochi, fruit, nuts

Special Food Tips

Mochi is made from pounded rice. You can find it in the refrigerated section in health food stores. Cut it into 1-inch squares and bake for 10 minutes in a toaster oven.

Crock-Pot Recipe: Purchase a quart-size Crock-Pot. Just before bed, measure out 3 to 4 ounces of three grains and seeds. (Have on hand: organic rye, kamut, quinoa, millet, barley, oats, sunflower seeds, and pumpkin seeds—rotate them through the week.) Cover with 10 to 12 ounces of water and plug in overnight. In the morning you have a delicious cooked cereal. If it's too dry, add hot water and stir. Eat with fruit and two tablespoons of flaxseed oil.

Weekend Cooking Spree

Here's what I do to have food on hand for the week. Place one or two fresh or frozen (free-range) chickens in a big stockpot on top of a regular vegetable steamer tray. Add two tablespoons of curry to the water. Keep about one quart of water on a slow to medium boil, and steam. If you start with frozen chickens, cook for just over one hour—then check to see if the leg pulls away with pink but not blood showing at the bone, at which point you can add whole organic yams, beets, and onions—you don't even have to cut them up. At the 1½ hour mark, add whole potatoes. At the 1¾ hour mark, add whole carrots and cut-up squash. In the final 5 minutes, add greens (kale, collards, spinach). It may take two hours to cook but it only requires a few minutes of prep time. (For fresh chickens the cooking time is about ½ hour less.)

Your first meal is a nice chicken dinner with all the trimmings. The rest you can freeze, including the quart of chicken stock, or you can immediately make a soup with the rest of the leftovers. Start by cooking rice in the chicken stock. Use basmati for an interesting taste. Then add some of the cooked chicken and all the vegetables.

You can add coconut milk, more curry to taste, and any frozen vegetables you have on hand. I make 6 quarts at a time, freezing some and eating the rest over the next two days.

Focus on Fiber

If constipation is a constant companion, you need to add fiber to your diet. You can purchase several types of fiber: wheat bran, oat bran, or rice bran. Take one to three tablespoons on your cereal, or mixed in juice, your greens drink, or your balanced nutrition product. Make sure to drink extra water along with the bran. Actually, an extra few glasses of water a day will greatly help with constipation. By following the Menopause Diet you will be eating more vegetables, whole grains, nuts, and seeds, which are loaded with fiber. In fact, you may find yourself getting more gas as your intestinal flora gets used to your new regimen.

Beyond bran, you can use psyllium seed powder. The dosage is two teaspoons shaken in eight ounces of water and then an additional eight ounces of water is taken; this is done twice a day. A little juice can be added for taste. You can also purchase psyllium seed capsules and take three or four twice a day along with several glasses of water. If you use psyllium and do not use extra water, you can actually cause constipation. One general note about bran and psyllium is that they should be taken away from meals so that nutrients are not bound to the fiber and pulled out of the body.

The mineral that is a natural laxative and should be on any woman's supplement list is magnesium.

Exercise for Menopause

Daily exercise is important at any age. From thirty minutes to an hour is optimal. You can break up your exercise into several parts—

walking, free weights, and aerobic. Exercise is beneficial for bones, heart, mood, and weight, the four things we worry about most as we age.

I used to do yoga every day and get in a long walk but I knew I should also be using free weights to put more emphasis on bone building. Then my friend Dr. Margaret Merrifield told me she was advising her patients to do an exercise program called T-Tapp. Since she is also my doctor, I took it as a prescription and sent away for a couple of DVDs and have been doing it while writing *Hormone Balance*. I love it. I do a walking sequence and a basic workout sequence. I alternate them every day and after I exercise I feel energized and ready to go back to writing.

Most exercises work only one part of a muscle, steadily building up layers of short bulky muscle fiber. After learning about T-Tapp, I realized how short-sighted this approach is. By contrast, the T-Tapp technique works the whole length of each muscle, creating long smooth muscle fibers. Holding the T-Tapp body position while doing the exercises engages at least five muscles at once. T-Tapp moves are also designed to stimulate the body's nerve pathways. By receiving full nerve stimulation, muscle fibers contract more fully and therefore become firmer more quickly, directly impacting metabolism.

Muscle tissue requires ten times more calories to sustain itself than any other type of body tissue. Studies show that adding five pounds of taut muscle increases your calorie-burning power by 200 calories per day—even on days when you don't exercise. Just having the extra muscle bulk burns calories; they're looking for fuel, and they'll use body fat to get it. Therese Tapp says, "[I]t's common to lose inches two to three times faster with T-Tapp than with other types of exercises." She says it's as much about losing inches as losing weight, because you may add muscle weight while losing fat and losing inches.

Another factor that was important to me about T-Tapp exercise is the power to control blood sugar. I've said many times how important it is to control blood sugar and prevent insulin surges— excess sugar is shunted into fat storage by insulin. Avoiding excess sugar in the blood means less fat goes into storage. Theresa says that people with diabetes and high blood sugar have been able to normalize their blood sugar levels with regular exercise, probably by burning large amounts of calories.

In her April 2004 newsletter, Theresa says that she designed her workouts to be much more than a system to burn calories and fat. It does that very well but she knew she could create a system that would "rebuild primary body functions such as digestion, assimilation and elimination, as well as lymphatic and neuro-kinetic flow. The special sequence of these movements also stimulates release of several neuro-transmitters, hormones and other biochemical factors involved in metabolic homeostasis."

My Personal T-Tapp

My personal experience with T-Tapp after just a few weeks is very positive. I stand up straighter, feel stronger, am developing visible triceps, and now know why I can't do side bends. Teresa identifies people as having short torsos and long torsos. I have a short torso, therefore, my ribs hit my hips when I do side bends, making it impossible for me to do anything more than a token bend to the side.

Learning from Teresa how to walk with my feet pointed forward and not in a slight duck walk will also save my hips and a lot of grief in the future. People who do an exaggerated duck walk (think ballerinas) will run into trouble because they are putting undue pressure on their hip joints thousands of times a day!

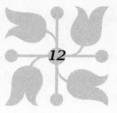

12

Natural Hormonal Supplements

ALTHOUGH SOME FOLKS may dive into this chapter thinking that taking a few supplements is the answer to hormonal balance problems, I want to remind you that diet and exercise will give you a very solid foundation and form the basis of any wellness program. So don't forget to read Chapter 11 on diet and exercise.

✐ Jumping Ship

There is widespread controversy as to how women on HRT should respond to the Women's Health Initiative study that showed ERT and HRT to be unsafe. One survey, by the Kaiser Foundation, found that 25 percent of women who stopped HRT because of the news resumed lower dose HRT because of hot flashes and night sweats that disturbed their sleep. However, that leaves 75 percent of women who stayed off HRT and might not have needed hormone replacement in the first place. It seems to me that that percentage probably represents an incredible number of women who were taking a potentially dangerous and unnecessary drug.

Actually, going off HRT in this way is what we in medicine call "taking a drug holiday." It's not unusual for people to find themselves taking a number of conflicting medications. To sort out what is necessary and what is not, doctors will cut out all but the most crucial ones and monitor symptoms to see which ones you really need. That is happening with HRT. By going off the pills, many women are either finding that they don't need them—they can put up with the symptoms—or finding natural solutions for menopausal complaints.

Taper Your Drugs

It may be better, however, to taper your dosage. Ask your doctor for a lower dose pill so that you can take half your usual dosage for a few weeks, then one-quarter of the dosage, while at the same time following the diet and supplement program that I'm recommending.

⚘ The Safety of Supplements

We've been scientifically studying vitamins for over sixty years—enough time to prove beyond a shadow of a doubt their safety and efficacy. Herbs have been used for centuries by cultures around the world without ill effects. Many people, however, are confused when they see lurid headlines about the dangers of vitamins and herbs. What are we to think?

You may not realize that there is a battle on the supplement front. News that the herb ephedra was responsible for several deaths caused an explosion of stories in the media in 2003 resulting in an ephedra ban. When used properly—in combination with other herbs, and at low doses—ephedra is a treatment for asthma. In fact, many over-the-counter drugs contain a synthetic form of ephedra, still on the shelves waiting to be abused. A negative combination of unscrupulous manufacturers producing high-potency ephedra products for weight loss and a gullible public taking pills above the recommended dosage resulted in dangerous side effects. The solution is not to ban the herb but to educate both manufacturers and consumers in the wise use of herbs. In April 2005, the ban was lifted.

It seems that drug companies feel they should control the vitamin and herb market and they are pressuring the government to put restrictions on supplements, ban high-dose products, and make supplements prescription items. That way supplements may only be produced by licensed pharmaceutical companies. To find out more about this you can research Codex Alimentarius, the World Trade Organization's committee to institute worldwide standards on food and supplements. (Resource: Friends of Freedom *www.friendsof freedom.org* and The National Health Federation *www.thenhf.com*)

The *Journal of Orthomolecular Medicine* published an editorial by renowned psychiatrist Dr. Abram Hoffer in May 2003 about toxic vitamins. Dr. Hoffer reminds us that forty years ago, vitamin researchers concluded that

- Vitamins are needed only in very small amounts, as declared by the recommended daily allowance (RDA).
- They are used only to prevent certain classical deficiency diseases. Thiamine prevents beri beri, vitamin C prevents scurvy, vitamin D prevents rickets, and vitamin B_3 prevents pellagra.

Surprisingly, most doctors still cling to these two very old notions that I learned in medical school. In the meantime, we have discovered that all processes in the body require cofactors and these cofactors are vitamins and minerals. Keying in fifty known nutrients in a medical publication data bank turns up almost half a million studies on these nutrients.

We now know the following about vitamins, minerals, and herbs:

- Homocysteine disease requires B_6, B_{12}, folic acid, and magnesium to protect the heart.
- Niacin in high doses is an excellent treatment for high cholesterol.
- Vitamin E is a treatment for heart disease.
- Vitamin C in high doses treats a wide variety of infectious diseases and cancer.
- Niacinamide is used in the treatment of some forms of arthritis.
- Antioxidants delay the onset and severity of Alzheimer's disease.
- Antioxidants prevent some forms of cancer.
- Magnesium prevents heart disease and twenty-two other conditions.
- Mild to moderate depression can be treated with Saint John's wort.
- Menopause symptoms can be treated with red clover and black cohosh.
- The immune system responds positively to treatment with echinacea, garlic, and astragalus.

However, in spite of thousands of reports to the contrary, many doctors still believe what they learned in medical school—to the detriment of their patients and public health. Considering their doctors to be the authorities on health matters, patients often believe their doctor when he or she says, "You can get all the vitamins from your food; don't waste your money." Let me remind you, doctors learn very little about the therapeutic use of nutrients. I had to study naturopathic medicine and earn a degree to learn about the proper use of nutrients.

Doctors learn about disease and drugs and when to refer to specialists. They don't learn about wellness. To top it all off, doctors are very reluctant to admit that they don't know something. So instead of saying that they don't know about nutrients and referring patients to someone who does, they claim that supplements are not necessary—or even that they're a waste of money. Doctors also assume that if it is worth knowing they would have learned about it in medical school, so they go out of their way to declare vitamins—especially in high doses—not only contraindicated by dangerous. A 2004 survey of people using complementary alternative medicine found that "27.7% of individuals who use CAM believed that conventional medicine would not help their health care problem. These data are contrary to a previous observation that CAM users are not, in general, dissatisfied with conventional medicine." (Barnes, P.; Powell-Griner, E.; McFann, K.; Nahin, R. *CDC Advance Data Report #343.* Complementary and Alternative Medicine Use among Adults: United States. May 27, 2004.) It's a matter of trust, and often, that trust is eroded when a patient has had great benefit from a nutrient yet their doctor denies its worth. Vitamins may also be required in greater amounts because of our highly polluted environment.

Many vitamins, minerals, and herbs act as antioxidants to protect the DNA of our cells from the damage caused by free radicals and mutagens. They prevent harmful genetic alterations within cells and chromosomes. Antioxidants are especially important with our current level of environmental pollution because they combat the effects of many toxins such as ozone, carbon monoxide, hydrocarbons, pesticides, heavy metals, nitrates, and industrial chemicals numbering in the thousands.

✺ Menopause-Friendly Nutrients

This notion of using supplements for health and to prevent disease has been evolving over the past few decades. I remember as a kid being given cod liver oil, and that was about it. I don't think my mother took vitamins at all. Now, as we recognize the side effects of drugs and we see the benefits of supplements, there are many nutrients and families of nutrients that we can turn to.

- Isoflavones
- Herbs: red clover, black cohosh, dong quai
- Vitamins
- Minerals
- DHEA

✐ Phytoestrogens

Dr. Tori Hudson wrote an overview of alternatives to HRT in *The Townsend Letter*, November 2002. In it, she explained that phytoestrogens cannot act in the same negative way that estrogens do because they selectively bind to a particular form of the estrogen receptor, which directs their positive effects toward the central nervous system, blood vessels, bones, and skin. That means they do not bind to receptors that cause stimulation of the breast or uterus.

Isoflavones at Work

The potency of soy isoflavones is 400 to 1,000 times less than estradiol. As mentioned earlier, isoflavones are said to act as weak estrogens helping to relieve menopausal symptoms while apparently blocking harmful estrogenic compounds, and decreasing uterine and breast cancer risk. Isoflavones are also promoted as cholesterol-lowering agents. They may also promote bone health by increasing bone density in menopause through a combination of inhibiting bone deterioration and stimulating bone formation.

Over the past decade there has been a scientific tennis game played with isoflavones as the ball. First, one study says isoflavones help menopausal symptoms; the next one says they don't. The most recent tally is that they may, indeed, help menopausal symptoms, but at a high price. Studies in two journals *Fertility & Sterility* and the *Journal of the American Medical Association*, both published in July 2004, concluded that soy supplements containing isoflavones do not help lower cholesterol, or boost bone density, or keep the mind sharp after menopause, and may even cause cancer. These recent findings support my caution about using processed soy or soy supplements on a regular basis for menopause symptoms.

No More Red Faces with Red Clover—Trifolium pratens

You can sprout red clover seeds or find them in supplement form, or you can go to a farm and see red clover being used to feed the animals. I haven't tried red clover yet—I mean the supplements, not the hay—but I'm sure I will. I like to rotate supplements so my body doesn't get bored with them and not "listen" anymore. Clinical trials to determine the efficacy of red clover have much the same track record as that of the isoflavones but with a two-to-one score in favor of red clover.

Dosage for red clover: Tincture: 30 to 60 drops, three times per day. Capsules: 500 mg, 2–6 per day.

Beating Menopause with Black Cohosh—Cimicifuga racemosa

Black cohosh has been used for relief of menopausal symptoms by Native Americans, possibly for thousands of years. Knowledge of the many uses of this plant was passed on to early settlers. It is one of the few herbs that can relieve vaginal dryness because of its mild estrogenic effects. It also tames hot flashes, and is a muscle and nerve relaxant to the extent that it reduces menopausal depression. It alleviates arthritic pains, improves digestion, and strengthens the pelvic muscles and thus helps prevent prolapse. The beneficial effects of black cohosh don't stop there. Regarding heart and blood vessels, it dilates blood vessels and thins the blood, thereby increasing circulation and lowering blood pressure. The focus of recent research has turned toward its anticancer properties. A 1998 review of eight clinical trials of black cohosh found that it is a safe and effective alternative to ERT and can be safely used by women who should not use ERT.[37] Dr. Tori Hudson says it's considered a suitable natural alternative to HRT, especially for women at high risk for cancer.

Even though black cohosh has passed the test of time and the test of scientific research, I still see researchers battling out which herbal preparation is best for menopause. Black cohosh has been studied as a stand-alone supplement, and it works quite well that way, but I suspect black cohosh works better in combination with other herbs. That's the way I was trained in herbal medicine. Combine plants that have similar actions to boost their effects. Therefore, you might find that a combination of herbs along with black cohosh works best for you. Such a combination might include motherwort, ginseng, evening primrose oil, burdock root, licorice root, red raspberry leaves, dong quoi, sarsaparilla, wild yam, spearmint, damiana, motherwort, or vitex (chasteberry). See below for more details on these herbs. There may not be studies on such combinations, but you can select a high-end product and do your own individual research study. By high end, I mean don't buy the cheapest herbal product on the shelf. Cheapness means low-quality herbs—the dregs that are left on the sorting floor after the high-quality parts have been stripped. Legally they are still herbs, but may just be the stems instead of the flowering tops or the deep roots that you think you're getting.

Dosage for black cohosh: Tincture: 10–30 drops a day. Capsules: 500 mg, one to three times per day. Standardized extract capsules: 20 mg, 2 per day.

Doing Dang Quoi—Angelica sinensis

Dang quoi is a "female" herb, high in phytoestrogens, for all stages in a woman's life—for pregnancy and delivery, perimenopause, and menopause. Dang quoi relieves hot flashes, but it works better for stressed women who suffer hot flashes but are generally chilly. It's a nourishing herb containing many nutrients that works part of its magic by supporting the liver. It increases vaginal secretions as well as stimulating circulation to the face to convey a healthy glow. Dang quoi thins the blood, and Chinese practitioners use it instead of aspirin, without the side effects. It lessens heart palpitations, lowers blood pressure, and increases the circulation to prevent heart disease. It also relieves insomnia, joint pain, and nervous tension, common symptoms in menopause.

Dosage for dang quoi: Tincture: 10–40 drops of dang quoi root one to three times a day. Capsules: 500 mg, 2–3 per day.

Cautions: Don't use if you are taking aspirin. Don't use if you have heavy bleeding or fibroids; because dang quoi increases circulation, it could increase bleeding. Stop if you get breast tenderness.

Going with Ginseng

When I was in practice, wild Red Korean Ginseng was the herb of choice for menopause. It's a "male" herb used as a tonic for potency, stress, and energy and only used by women after menopause. Red Korean is simply the commonly known white Chinese ginseng, grown in Korea, harvested, and dried in the sun, which changes its color. Over the past decade, studies on the herbs mentioned above have eclipsed ginseng. However, it is still a fine herb that is used either alone or in formulas. Part of the reason it is not in common usage may simply be that the wild form is almost extinct and ridiculously expensive. Cultivated ginseng is the form that you will find in usage today.

For menopause, ginseng is a tonic for the adrenals, liver, nervous system, and immune system. It can prevent vaginal atrophy by increasing lubrication and preventing thinning of the vaginal lining. It is a common ingredient in formulas given for infertility and anovulatory cycles. It also supports detoxification, protects against X-ray radiation, and has anticancer activity.

Dosage for ginseng: Standardized extracts of ginsenosides—look for 4 to 6 percent ginsenosides and take 100 mg twice per day. Non-standardized root powder or extracts—take 1–2 grams daily. Chinese herbalists recommend this herb only be taken for two months at a time with a one-month rest before resuming. If used in smaller amounts in a complex formula, you would not have to follow this precaution.

A Word about Wild Yam

Wild yam is a rich source of diosgenin, a natural precursor to progesterone and other phytoestrogens. It is effective for many symptoms of menopause and often used in natural hormone replacement formulas in tincture or capsule form. Wild yam creams have the ability to restore vaginal moistness and elasticity as well as being used as a symptom preventative and to decrease risk of osteoporosis. The recommended dosage is 10–30 drops tincture daily.

There is an ongoing debate about using wild yam creams as a source of progesterone. The confusion comes because some companies put the actual drug, progesterone USP (United States Pharmacopeial Convention—a body that standardizes drugs) in their wild yam creams and some don't. The ones that contain progesterone have a direct progesterone effect. The creams that don't contain progesterone USP just have the effect of the plant. Not all wild yam creams are created equally—check the label and check with the supplier. If you take a wild yam cream that contains progesterone, you should have your progesterone levels checked every six to twelve months. See Chapter 13 for more on hormone testing.

✕ Herbal Combinations for Menopause

Many herbalists feel that taking one herb, on its own, for long periods of time may cause side effects. These effects can be attenuated by using a combination of synergistic herbs. When conventional medicine takes herbal prescribing a step backward by isolating the most active ingredient and then making it out of synthetic chemicals, you are bound to get side effects. Herbal formulas for menopause often contain the following herbs, which are used in capsule or tincture form. The major ingredients may be black cohosh, dang quoi, or red clover, and the associated herbs either support their action or can function on their own.

- Blue vervain is an important herb for the nervous system. It calms the mood, relieving irritability and insomnia.
- Elderberry contains bioflavins and anti-inflammatories that improve circulation and decrease joint pain.
- False unicorn contains phytosterols (plant steroids), making it useful in balancing hormones and controlling hot flashes; in early menopause, it is used to control heavy bleeding.
- Fenugreek contains phytosterols and is used for hot flashes.
- Licorice root contains substances similar to the natural steroids of the body and thereby supports the hormonal system and stimulates adrenal gland production. It should not be used as a single herb because in large amounts it can increase blood pressure.
- Motherwort relieves hot flashes, anxiety, insomnia, and palpitations, and strengthens vaginal tissue.
- Nettles restore and strengthen kidney and adrenal function, have a high mineral content, stabilize blood sugar, and relieve joint pain.
- Red raspberry leaves strengthen and tone the muscles of the uterus.

- Sage helps eliminate hot flashes, night sweats, mood changes, headaches, indigestion, and joint aches.
- Sarsaparilla contains substances that stimulate progesterone activity in the body.
- Saint John's wort has been proven to relieve mild to moderate depression.

✣ Vitamins and Minerals

While researching *The Miracle of Magnesium*, I developed a new respect for these simple nutrients that make everything happen in the body. They are the cofactors for every metabolic process; without them, nothing would happen in the body. Modern medicine pays so little attention to these nutrients that they are processed out of all packaged foods. Attempts to "fortify" foods with nutrients means that a fraction of the various nutrients is replaced, all in synthetic forms that the body may easily reject. Doctors who say we get all the nutrients we need from our diet or fortified foods still believe their medical school training where they were taught that only a small amount of vitamins are needed to prevent deficiency diseases such as scurvy (vitamin C), beri beri (vitamin B_1), or pellagra (vitamin B_3). Now we know that the B vitamins are crucial to prevent homocysteinuria that causes heart disease; magnesium is necessary for bone formation and a healthy heart; and vitamin B_3 (niacin) treats high cholesterol.

✣ The B Complex Vitamins

The B vitamins are cofactors in the production and metabolism of hormones. They are essential for healthy brain and nerve function and for energy production. They help reduce menopause-related depression, anxiety, and fatigue. They also assist in protein and fat metabolism while normalizing blood sugar levels. The recommended dosage by alternative medicine practitioners is 50–100 milligrams daily taken in divided doses, which is much higher than the ridiculously low amounts in the government RDAs.

B vitamins are water-soluble and don't build up in the body, so they are extremely safe. Vitamin B_6 is depleted by the birth control pill. In fact, most drugs will cause depletion of vitamins and minerals that are cofactors in metabolizing and detoxifying foreign chemicals.

One counterargument to doctors who say that taking vitamins will just give you expensive urine is this: Vitamins in the bladder are still at work! And you have had to take enough for them to come out in the urine. Food sources for the individual B vitamins are listed below; however, even though whole grains are good sources of most of the B vitamins, processing and refining grains may result in 75 percent loss of these nutrients.

Vitamin B_1

This vitamin, also called thiamine, functions in carbohydrate metabolism to help convert food into energy. It also helps maintain the nervous system, memory, and heart muscle health.

A deficiency of thiamine causes a condition known as beri beri. In North America, thiamine deficiency is said to be most common in alcoholics and people who are malnourished. It is likely that many people are malnourished and deficient in vitamin B_1 and don't even realize it. By knowing its deficiency symptoms, you can see how important vitamin B_1 is for the body. You may also see some of your own symptoms in this list, indicating a special need that you may have for this B vitamin.

The major deficiency symptoms affect the nervous system and heart causing the following.

- Sensory disturbances
- Muscle weakness
- Impaired memory

- Shortness of breath
- Palpitation
- Eventual heart failure

Scientific research shows that the more you eat, the more vitamin B_1 you need to process your food. It's not just people who overeat who create a vitamin B_1 deficiency but also athletes who consume more calories for their high-energy workouts. Stress also puts more demand on vitamin B_1—as it does on all the nutrients in your body.

Sources: Nuts, liver, brewer's yeast

Dosage: Even though the RDA is a few milligrams per day, it is advisable to take a vitamin B complex that has at least 25 mg of B_1, twice daily.

Vitamin B_2

Vitamin B_2, or riboflavin, is an important coenzyme for many metabolic processes in the body. It helps release energy from carbohydrates, fats, and proteins. It also helps to maintain the integrity of red blood cells and the nervous system. Studies show that it increases energy levels; can lessen the symptoms of chronic fatigue and improve concentration and mood. Like thiamine, riboflavin is involved in producing energy. People who become riboflavin-deficient may have a poor diet, chronic infections, liver disease, or alcoholism.

The signs and symptoms of riboflavin deficiency are the following:

- Sore throat
- Cracks, tears, or sores at the corners of your mouth
- Swollen tongue, seborrheic dermatitis, anemia, and impaired nerve function.

As with most B vitamins, the more food you eat, the more B vitamins you need to support the metabolic processes that will convert that food into usable energy. You need more riboflavin during pregnancy and breastfeeding. The birth control pill causes riboflavin wasting, and depletion of all the B vitamins. Athletes consuming extra calories require more riboflavin.

Sources: Liver, dairy products, dark green vegetables, and many types of seafood

Dosage: Even though the RDA is a few milligrams per day, it is advisable to take a vitamin B complex that has at least 25 mg of B_2, twice daily.

Side Effects: The only effect of riboflavin is a bright yellow color to the urine. Some practitioners say that if you take a B vitamin complex and your urine does not turn yellow, then you may need more.

Vitamin B_3

Vitamin B_3—also called niacin, inositol hexaniacinate, niacinamide, and nicotinic acid—is another water-soluble B vitamin. Niacin is involved in many aspects of energy metabolism and nervous system function. It's the vitamin that you can give to your family, in a dosage of about 100 milligrams, to show them what a hot flash is really like! However, some people may get a skin flush from only 25 milligrams.

Niacin has a role to play in more than 200 enzyme systems that release energy from carbohydrates and fats, metabolize proteins, make certain hormones, and assist in the formation of red blood cells. Current research confirms that niacin lowers cholesterol and triglycerides; it may also prevent and treat diabetes (as niacinamide); improve circulation (as inositol hexaniacinate); and relieve arthritis (as niacinamide).

Niacin deficiency symptoms mostly affect the skin, nervous system, and gastrointestinal tract. They include:

- Skin rash
- Headache
- Depression
- Impaired memory
- Hallucinations
- Dementia
- Diarrhea, nausea, vomiting
- Swollen tongue

Sources: Meat, chicken, tuna and other fatty fish, peanuts, pork, and milk

Dosage: The RDA for niacin, to avoid frank deficiency, is only 13–18 mg. The cholesterol-lowering dose of niacin (as nicotinic acid) is typically in the range of 250–2,000 mg/day. Dosing is usually started at the low end (250 mg/day) with increasing doses of 250 mg each week or two until blood lipid levels start to normalize (or side effects develop). For daily supplement needs, 50 mg once or twice per day in a vitamin B complex is my usual recommendation.

Side Effects: With high doses used for controlling cholesterol levels—anything above 100 mg/day—nicotinic acid can cause skin flushing and itching of the skin as well as headaches and hypotension (lightheadedness and low blood pressure).

Vitamin B$_5$

Vitamin B$_5$ is also called pantothenic acid. It is a precursor to Coenzyme A, an essential enzyme for the metabolism of carbohydrates, the synthesis and degradation of fats, and the synthesis of sterols, which produce steroid hormones including melatonin. Vitamin B$_5$ is also important for the synthesis of the neurotransmitter acetylcholine and heme, a component of hemoglobin. Detoxification of many drugs and toxins requires CoA in the liver.

Vitamin B_5 is the vitamin that Dr. Margaret Merrifield recommends for her "burnt-out" patients. She finds that women with low adrenal function improve greatly with the use of 1,000 mg of vitamin B_5 once or twice per day. As you can see above, it is necessary for the production of hormones, including adrenal hormones.

At the Linus Pauling Institute, experiments on vitamin B_5–deficient animals gave the following results: rats showed damaged adrenal glands; monkeys developed anemia, low blood sugar, rapid breathing, rapid heart rates, and convulsions; chickens developed spinal nerve damage associated with the degeneration of the myelin sheath, skin irritation, and feather abnormalities; mice showed decreased exercise tolerance and diminished storage of glucose (in the form of glycogen) in muscle and liver and also developed skin irritation and graying of the fur.

Currently known symptoms of vitamin B_5 deficiency in humans include:

- Numbness and painful burning and tingling of the feet
- Headache
- Fatigue
- Insomnia
- Intestinal disturbances

Source: Liver and kidney, yeast, egg yolk, and broccoli

Dosage: The Food and Nutrition Board of the Institute of Medicine—which operates on the "vitamins as prevention of frank deficiency model"—reports that there is insufficient evidence to establish RDAs for pantothenic acid, and it set "adequate intake levels" ranging from 1.7 to 7 milligrams per day. I recommend at least 50 milligrams of B_5 twice daily as a general supplement. However, for adrenal deficiency I recommend much larger doses. When I am under stress, I personally take 1,000 milligrams once or twice daily in a powder form with protein powder, my Green Drink, or freshly prepared vegetable juice. There are many green drinks presently on the market. They consist of a variety of vegetable, fruits, sprouted grains, and herbs dried and powdered that you can easily dissolve in water or diluted fruit juice to help get your daily quota of vegetables and fruits.

Side Effects: There are no reported side effects for vitamin B_5, even in high doses.

Vitamin B_6

Vitamin B_6 is also called pyridoxine. It is essential for the proper function of over seventy different enzymes in the body. Vitamin B_6 participates in amino acid metabolism to create protein and carbohydrate and fat metabolism. It also helps synthesize neurotransmitters in the brain involved in nerve conduction, supports mental function, and improves emotional outlook and mood through serotonin synthesis. B_6 is necessary for hemoglobin synthesis and red blood cell growth, and immune support (white blood cell development). Many integrative medicine specialists recommend high doses of vitamin B_6 for the relief of arthritis.

Vitamin B_6 is needed in higher amounts if you are on a high-protein diet. The latest high-protein diet fad is bound to produce symptoms of vitamin B_6 deficiency. The birth control pill also causes a demand for higher amounts of this vitamin. Vitamin B_6 has achieved a certain positive notoriety in the past few years because it, along with folic acid and vitamin B_{12}, is a treatment for excess homocysteine, which causes heart disease. It is also necessary in the conversion of the amino acid tryptophan into niacin, and therefore is involved in lowering cholesterol.

Vitamin B_6 plays a role in prostaglandin synthesis, which is the body's natural anti-inflammatory. Therefore, it is used for pain, carpal tunnel syndrome, inflammation, and PMS. It has diuretic effects that help regulate blood pressure and heart function. Combined with magnesium, vitamin B_6 reduces oxalate excretion and decreases the occurrence of kidney stones. Clinical trials have shown it to be a useful adjunctive treatment for autism.

Deficiency symptoms include:

- Seborrhea, a skin condition that produces dry, flaky lesions around the eyes, nose and mouth
- Sores in the mouth and on the tongue
- Depression
- Irritability
- Confusion

Sources: Poultry, fish, whole grains, and bananas

Dosage: Although the RDA for vitamin B_6 is a mere 2 mg, I recommend 25–50 mg per day. The dosage for relieving PMS and carpal tunnel and treating kidney stones may be 100 mg one to three times per day.

Side Effects: As a water-soluble B vitamin, B_6 is generally very safe as a dietary supplement. When taken in excessive intakes, 2,000–6,000 mg daily for several months, there have been reports of numbness in the extremities, which may or may not be reversible.

Vitamin B_9—Folic Acid

Folic acid is rarely called vitamin B_9, but that is its numerical designation. Folic acid is extremely important in the synthesis of components of DNA and RNA. Adequate intake can reduce damage to DNA and deficiency can cause damage. It is also necessary for normal red blood cell formation, and deficiency can lead to one form of anemia that is difficult to distinguish from vitamin B_{12} deficiency.

Folic acid deficiency causes neural tube birth defects; it is essential during preconception and pregnancy. The BCP causes folic acid deficiency and may result in birth defects if women become pregnant soon after stopping the pill. Most American women of childbearing age have folic acid intakes below the recommended 400 micrograms per day. The elderly are also at increased risk for folate deficiencies, which may exacerbate the risk of neurological disease, heart disease, and cancer that are more prevalent in this population.

Several recent studies have suggested that folate supplementation should be given to elderly people, especially those with elevated plasma total homocysteine levels and cardiovascular disease, as well as in those individuals who experience neuropsychiatric disorders.

Folic acid deficiency is common in people who have Crohn's disease. The small intestine is often a focus of damage in Crohn's as well as the site where folic acid is absorbed from food. Excessive intake of alcohol can also result in folic acid deficiency. Folic acid function can be hampered by several drugs, including nonsteroidal anti-inflammatory drugs (NSAIDs), methotrexate (cancer chemotherapy), trimethoprim (an antibiotic), cholestyramine (a cholesterol drug), isoniazid (a TB drug), and triamterene (a diuretic).

Deficiency symptoms include:

- Sore mouth
- Sore tongue
- Weakness
- Irritability
- Numbness and tingling in the hands and feet
- Seizures

Sources: Fruits, dark leafy greens, oranges and orange juice, beans and peas, and brewer's yeast

Dosage: The RDA for folic acid for adults over thirteen years is 400 micrograms; for pregnant women, 600 micrograms; and for lactating women, 500 micrograms. It is also recommended that the elderly receive 500 micrograms a day. I recommend 1,000 micrograms per day of folic acid along with 100 milligrams per day of vitamin B_{12}.

Side Effects: The only side effect of folic acid and the reason you have to get high doses on prescription is that high intakes (1–5 mg/day) have been associated with masking the signs and symptoms of pernicious anemia, which is a vitamin B_{12} deficiency. The simple solution is to take folic acid along with vitamin B_{12}.

Vitamin B_{12}

Vitamin B_{12} is a water-soluble, cobalt-containing nutrient in the vitamin B complex family. Along with most of the other B vitamins, it is a cofactor in enzymes involved in the metabolism of proteins, fats, and carbohydrates; and energy; and, along with folic acid and vitamin B_6, it controls homocysteine levels, which elevate the risk of heart disease. Vitamin B_{12} is also a necessary component in the synthesis of the insulating myelin sheath around neurons, for cell reproduction, and for proper red blood cell production. B_{12} is required for the rapid synthesis of DNA during cell division. This is especially true for red blood cell formation, where new cells are formed daily and a whole new blood supply is formed in about three months. B_{12} deficiency produces the characteristic signs of abnormal red blood cells and a form of anemia called pernicious anemia.

Deficiency of vitamin B_{12} occurs mostly in vegetarians and in people who have absorption problems. B_{12} requires "intrinsic factor," which is secreted by the stomach, to properly absorb B_{12} into the small intestine. A lack of intrinsic factor or intestinal disease such as Crohn's necessitates vitamin B_{12} injections on a regular basis.

Deficiency symptoms of vitamin B_{12} include:

- Generalized fatigue and exhaustion
- Shortness of breath
- Listlessness
- Paleness
- Increased risk of infection

- Sore tongue
- Anemia
- Nerve tingling

Source: Primarily found in animal products: meat, eggs, and dairy products. B_{12} is most beneficial when given by injection and is poorly absorbed orally. Sublingual tablets that are absorbed under the tongue may bypass the need for intrinsic factor in the stomach. However, more research needs to be done on B_{12}, since it plays an important role in preventing heart disease, neurological disease, and aging. Studies of people with homocysteine elevation, dementia, and Alzheimer's consistently show low levels of vitamin B_{12}.

Dosage: The RDA for vitamin B_{12} for adults is set at a very low 2.4 micrograms. The dosage that I recommend is 100 micrograms per day orally or 1,000 micrograms by injection once every two weeks.

Side Effects: There are no side effects from taking B_{12}.

Vitamin E

Vitamin E is a fat-soluble vitamin that makes up a family of eight related compounds known as tocopherols and tocotrienols. Vitamin E was discovered in the early 1930s. Rats on a vegetable oil-deficient diet became infertile. The cause was traced to a lack of vitamin E, which is mainly found in vegetable oil. Vitamin E is a powerful anti-oxidant that protects the heart from damage. The Shute brothers, two doctors in Ontario, Canada, proved the benefits of vitamin E on the heart in the 1950s.

Vitamin E also improves the circulation, supports the liver, and helps lubricate drying vaginal tissue. Several studies have shown that it can decrease menopausal hot flashes and improve overall health.

Sources: Vegetable oils, nuts, seeds, avocados, and wheat germ contain vitamin E in very small amounts.

Dosage: The RDA for vitamin E is only 15 to 22 IU to prevent frank heart damage from deficiency. However, most studies showing benefit for various health conditions use from 200 IU to 800 IU. The type of vitamin is also very important. Mixed tocopherols and tocotrienols are much more potent that just alpha-tocopherol, which is the most active form of vitamin E in humans. And the natural d-alpha-tocopherol is superior to the synthetic, dl-alpha tocopherols. Unfortunately, the synthetic "dl-" form is cheaper and is commonly found in dietary supplements.

Side Effects: Vitamin E is relatively nontoxic, even at very high doses of 1,000 to 2,000 IU.

Magnesium

The mineral magnesium functions as a coenzyme for over 325 enzymes in the body. It is responsible for cell, nerve, and muscle function; heart muscle and heart nerve conduction; regulation of body temperature: conversion of carbohydrates, protein, and fat into energy; DNA/RNA synthesis; and the formation of bones. Magnesium is the supplement of choice for menopause because it protects the heart, balances blood sugar, detoxifies the body, and slows the aging process.

Magnesium deficiency is widespread (about 80 percent of the population is deficient) due to lack of magnesium in the soil; destruction by food processing and cooking; and excessive requirements due to stress, drug toxicity, and generalized environmental toxicity.

Magnesium deficiency triggers or causes the following twenty conditions. Treating with magnesium can have a beneficial result.

- Anxiety and panic attacks
- Asthma
- Blood clots
- Bowel disease and constipation
- Cystitis and bladder spasms

- Depression
- Diabetes
- Fatigue
- Heart disease
- Hypertension
- Hypoglycemia
- Insomnia
- Kidney stones
- Migraine
- Musculoskeletal conditions: fibrositis, fibromyalgia, muscle spasms, eye twitching, cramps, and chronic neck and back pain
- Nerve problems: migraines; muscle contractions; gastrointestinal spasms; calf, foot, and toe cramps; vertigo; and confusion
- Obstetrics and gynecology: premenstrual syndrome, dysmenorrheal, infertility, premature contractions, preeclampsia and eclampsia of pregnancy
- Osteoporosis
- Raynaud's disease
- Sudden infant death syndrome
- Tooth decay
- Toxicity

Sources: Nuts, seeds, beans, and whole grains

Dosage: The RDA for magnesium is around 350 mg per day, an amount that most magnesium researchers find far too low to meet our needs. Two and three times that amount is advised. Magnesium oxide is only 40 percent absorbed, so it acts as a laxative; magnesium citrate is much better absorbed and therefore more effective; and magnesium glycinate does not have a laxative effect and can be used if you already have one or two bowel movements a day.

Side Effects: If you have too much magnesium you can get diarrhea—which is your indication to cut back. If you are on heart medications, you probably need extra magnesium, but be sure to discuss this with your doctor.

Manganese

Manganese is an essential trace mineral. It acts as a coenzyme for the antioxidant manganese superoxide dismutase (Mn SOD). Manganese acts as a necessary cofactor in the synthesis of fatty acids and cholesterol; mucopolysaccharide synthesis (in bones, collagen, and connective tissue); and glycoproteins, which coat body cells and protect against invading organisms. So, you can see how important it is for menopause—blood sugar balance, bones, joints, and immune system protection.

Sources: Tea, whole grains, nuts, and avocados

Dosage: The RDA is 1.4–5 mg. However, the amount for treating health conditions is about 5–10 mg per day.

Side Effects: There are few if any reported side effects of manganese.

Boron

Boron is a trace element associated with calcium and magnesium metabolism. Boron is concentrated in the bone, spleen, and thyroid, which gives an indication of boron's role in bone metabolism and suggesting a potential function for boron in hormone metabolism. Boron is useful in developing muscle mass; increasing muscle strength; maintaining strong bones; improving calcium absorption; and decreasing body fat—all very important functions for menopause. Interesting research shows that boron supplements can increase serum levels of testosterone in postmenopausal women and may help explain its benefits in menopause.

Sources: Nuts, dark green leafy vegetables, dried fruit, applesauce, grape juice, and beans and peas. Meat and fish are poor dietary sources of boron.

Dosage: There is no RDA set for boron. The therapeutic dosage ranges from 1 mg to 10 mg.

Side Effects: Neither boron nor its salt, boric acid, appears to have side effects at the recommended dosage.

Zinc

Zinc is an essential trace mineral that plays a role in more than 300 different enzymes in the body. Zinc is important for wound healing and immune system support; it reduces the length and severity of colds, prevents benign prostatic hyperplasia, and increases sperm production. More specifically for menopause, it enhances energy production, collagen synthesis, bone strength, cognitive function, digestion, and carbohydrate metabolism (glucose utilization and insulin production). Even mild zinc deficiency has been associated with depressed immunity, decreased sperm count, and impaired memory.

Sources: Seeds, seafood (especially oysters), meat, fish, eggs, poultry

Dosage: The adult RDA for zinc is 15 mg per day. Most people should take about 25 mg per day. Higher doses can reduce the copper levels in the body. Therapeutic zinc in higher doses should be followed by a health practitioner.

Side Effects: High doses of zinc—1,000 mg and higher—can cause nausea, diarrhea, and vomiting.

Vitamin C

Vitamin C, also known as ascorbic acid, is a water-soluble vitamin needed by the body for hundreds of vital metabolic reactions. We depend on our diet, or supplements, for vitamin C because it is not produced in the human body, yet it is essential for the formation of collagen, connective tissue, and immune system factors. Vitamin

C also has anti-inflammatory and antioxidant functions. Because it is required in the formation of collagen and connective tissue, vitamin C is necessary for building and maintaining strong bones, teeth, blood vessels, cartilage, tendons, and ligaments.

To counteract the increased risk of heart disease in menopause, vitamin C optimizes fat metabolism and protects tissues from free radical damage as an antioxidant. Vitamin C is a water-soluble antioxidant but it also helps restore vitamin E, which is a fat-soluble antioxidant.

Vitamin C deficiency causes scurvy, with bleeding gums, pain in the muscles and joints, skin lesions, fatigue, and bruising.

Sources: Citrus fruits (oranges, grapefruit, lemons), strawberries, tomatoes, broccoli, Brussels sprouts, peppers, and cantaloupe

Dosage: The absolute minimum amount of vitamin C necessary to prevent scurvy is about 10 mg. However, a daily dose of at least 100 mg is necessary for vitamin C to meet its requirements in the body. Most plants and animals are able to synthesize vitamin C for their needs. However, apes and humans cannot make it due to lack of an enzyme called gulonolactone oxidase.

Side Effects: Vitamin C is water-soluble and extremely safe. Even using ten grams a day, the only side effect will be loose bowel movement. Any claimed side effects such as increasing the incidence of kidney stones or increasing the absorption of iron have never been substantiated with actual clinical cases.

Vitamin D

Vitamin D is a fat-soluble vitamin produced in the skin and released into the blood to affect the bones. Its main function is to absorb and maintain adequate levels of calcium in the body. A feedback system with the parathyroid gland produces active vitamin D_3 when calcium levels are low. Vitamin D assists normal bone calcification by utilizing phosphorus and magnesium as well as calcium. Severe vitamin D deficiency results in rickets (in children) and osteomalacia (in adults); both of these are characterized by a reduced level of calcium being deposited in bones and a weakening of bone strength. Adequate vitamin D helps prevent osteoporosis.

Vitamin D is structurally related to estrogen and cortisone. Because it can be manufactured by the body through skin exposure to the sun, it is not classed as an essential nutrient. Vitamin D_2, or activated ergo-calciferol, is the major synthetic form of vitamin D. Vitamin D_3, or cholecalciferol, is found mainly in fish liver oils. These are converted in the liver and kidneys to 25-hydroxychole-calciferol and 1, 25-dihydroxylcholecalciferol, the major circulating active forms of vitamin D.

Sources: Vitamin D_3, or "natural" vitamin D, is found in fish liver oil, which is the traditional source of both A and D. Egg yolks, butter, and liver have some vitamin D, as do the oily fish, such as mackerel, salmon, sardines, and herring. Plant foods are fairly low in D, which means that strict vegetarians who are not exposed to fifteen minutes per day of sunlight do not get adequate amounts of vitamin D.

Dosage: The RDA for vitamin D is 400 IU per day.

Side Effects: Because vitamin D is a fat-soluble vitamin, it is stored in the body and has the potential to reach toxic levels if taken in high doses for prolonged periods of time. However, many researchers claim there are no side effects with intakes many times the RDA. Many people do not even achieve the RDA because of poor diets and lack of sunshine.

✕ DHEA

DHEA (dehydroepiandrosterone) is a hormone that is available over-the-counter in the United States. However, if you take it for menopause symptoms you should be under the care of a knowledgeable practitioner, and you should have blood or saliva tests to identify a deficiency and to follow your treatment. As women and men age, there appears to be a gradual decline in the level of DHEA in the blood. Blood levels become elevated with supplementation and subsequently increase the level of endorphins—the pain and pleasure neurotransmitters. Theoretically DHEA could have a positive effect on the mood swings of menopause. However, there is not enough research to confirm this theory. DHEA can also protect the heart, increase muscle tone and energy, and improve memory, all of which may be important for menopause.

DHEA is a precursor to estrogen and testosterone, which is another reason it should be taken under supervision. There is, however, a form of DHEA called 7-keto DHEA, a natural metabolite of DHEA, that is further down the pathway from estrogen and testosterone and does not produce these hormones.

⟋⁂ Traditional Medicine for Menopause

Homeopathy, acupuncture, acupressure, bioenergetics, Chinese medicine, massage, reiki, and dozens of other health modalities can have a place in the treatment of menopause. The best way to research these modalities is to ask your friends, your local health community workers, health food store owner, etc. People love to tell their health stories so it should not be too hard to find out who and what is helping people. Better yet, start a menopause support group where you can discuss treatments and invite local practitioners to give their views.

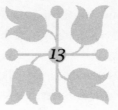

Bioidentical Hormones Versus Synthetic Hormones

BY NOW YOU HAVE SENSED my bias against synthetic hormones—partly because of the side effects and partly because I know there are so many natural alternatives. However, achieving hormonal balance is not just a matter of taking hormones in natural form. True balance is achieved by following a program of diet, exercise, supplements, and herbs, and then—if you need actual hormones—you have ones that are safer than synthetics.

Achieving Balance: Bioidentical Hormones

Natural hormones are not squeezed out of plants with your kitchen juicer, so they are not strictly natural. They go through a laboratory process to convert plant chemicals (soy and yam) into hormones that are bioidentical to the hormones produced in our bodies. Estradiol, estriol, estrone, progesterone, and testosterone can all be made by this process. Soy and yam are chosen because the chemical composition of one of their constituents is very close to the structure of hormones and can be converted to be biochemically identical to our body's sex hormones.

Natural/bioidentical hormones are prescribed, usually by integrative medicine practitioners, after assessment of your hormonal status with saliva or blood testing. We'll talk more about blood and saliva testing later in this chapter. The prescription often contains two or three estrogens—a bi-estrogen or tri-estrogen (estridiol and estriol or estrone, estradiol, and estriol) and may also contain progesterone, and occasionally testosterone. A compounding pharmacy makes up the formula, which is individualized to the patient's needs. Prescribing for the individual is far superior to the "one size fits all" method of synthetic hormone replacement. A word about compounding pharmacies: They often have a roster of doctors who use their services and may be willing to help you find a doctor who prescribes bioidentical hormones in your area.

⚘ Synthetic Hormones

Synthetic hormones are also produced in a lab but the starting molecules can be hydrocarbons—commonly called "coal tar derivatives"—and they are non-bioidentical. With the increasing demand for "natural" products, many synthetic hormones are now being derived from plant compounds—soy and yam—but have their chemical structure altered, making them non-bioidentical and patentable.

The pharmaceutical industry makes synthetic hormones non-bioidentical on purpose because you cannot patent a drug if it has the same molecular structure as a naturally occurring chemical in the body. Drug companies, however, can patent a synthetic drug that has a "similar" structure, and have a monopoly on the making and marketing of that drug for up to seventeen years. Drug companies may even say their drugs are plant-based or from natural sources to give the impression that they are just like your own hormones. But that is far from the truth. The underlying reason for making synthetic hormones is not for our benefit but because drugs must be synthetic to make a profit.

Patented drugs are not natural and the body cannot process them properly. For example, our body's naturally produced hormones and compounded bioidentical hormones are metabolized by the liver in approximately four hours, whereas synthetic hormones are partially metabolized and circulate in the body for over fourteen weeks.

It is true that synthetic hormones do have a "therapeutic" action on the body, but they also have a host of side effects that may include cancer. We have somehow come to accept that we have to take the bad with the good when it comes to drugs.

✎ Deconstructing Drugs

Natural, bioidentical; synthetic, non-bioidentical, conjugated, esterified—it's all very confusing. That's why many women just throw up their hands and let their doctor decide what they should take. However, your doctor may not know the ins and outs of bioidentical versus synthetic hormones. I certainly did not learn about natural, bioidentical hormones in medical school. Also, we have to remember that doctors have a difficult time accepting new treatments unless they are learned in medical school. Dr. Abram Hoffer, who has written twenty medical books and 500 scientific papers, has often stated that it takes about two generations before a truly new medical idea is accepted.

Let me give you a step-by-step introduction to hormones starting with the synthetics. Synthetic progesterone is called progestin; however, synthetic estrogen can still be called estrogen. Here is a list of different types of synthetic hormones available by prescription.

- Oral estrogen—conjugated
- Oral estrogen—plant-based
- Oral estrogen—esterified
- Skin patch estrogen—estradiol
- Cream estrogen—conjugated
- Ring estrogen
- Oral progestins
- Oral estrogen and progestin
- Skin patch-estrogen and progestin

Hormone Applications

Oral, skin patch, skin cream, and ring are the main forms of hormone therapy. Oral is by far the most common way of taking hormones, and skin patches are the second. I let out a big sigh when I think of all the doctors and drug companies that told patients not to worry about cortisone creams being absorbed. They had no idea how absorptive the skin really is. Now, there are a host of drugs delivered through skin patches, including hormones. Estrogen skin patches—Alora, Climara, FemPatch, and Vivelle—are all made from synthetic estradiol. Most patches are placed twice a week, on the abdomen or buttocks—avoiding the breasts, so there is no direct stimulation of breast tissue, and the waist, because movement of clothing might rub off the patch.

Absorption through the skin is more effective than taking estrogen by mouth. Taken by mouth, estrogen is absorbed into the bloodstream and travels through the liver where it is converted into weaker forms—as the body tries to get rid of the synthetic substance. Skin patches can contain three to ten times less estrogen than oral estrogen and achieve the same effect. Eventually, estrogen absorbed through the skin will reach the liver and be converted.

Estrogen creams are mostly designed to be used vaginally to increase vaginal lubrication and heal vaginal atrophy. A measured amount is squeezed into an applicator that is inserted into the vagina. Estrogen rings are less common, but serve the same function as vaginal creams. One brand is called Estring—a soft plastic ring that you or your doctor insert high into the vagina. Over the next ninety days, the ring releases estrogen. In the case of Estring the estrogen is estradiol.

What Are Conjugated Estrogens?

Premarin was the first estrogen available for commercial use; it is called a conjugated estrogen. Conjugated implies a mixture; in the case of Premarin, it is a mixture of water-soluble estrogens obtained from pregnant mares' urine—all its chemical constituents were not fully identified until fifty years after its first use. Conjugated estrogens USP is a standardized mixture only containing the main "ingredients" of mares' urine—estrone and equilin—or from estrogen prepared synthetically using estrone and equilin as the base. Synthetic conjugated estrogens contain a mix of nine different synthetic estrogens, allowing it to be patented. Very confusing and also very confusing for the body—having to detoxify nine chemicals every day.

Plant-Based Synthetic Estrogens

Plant-based estrogens (from soy and yam) have been made since the mid-1950s. The accompanying drug literature says that they "match the chemistry" of estrogen—usually estradiol, the most active estrogen and the one with the most side effects. Advertising promotes plant-based estrogens as being truly natural to the human female. They do not say these plant-based estrogens are bioidentical or match the molecular structure of estradiol. They are still synthetic, otherwise they would not be patented. Brands of plant-based estrogens include Climara, Estrace, Estraderm, Estring, Ogen, Ortho-Est, and Vivelle. In 1999, the FDA approved the first synthetic conjugated estrogen product called Cenestin. It mimics Premarin but is plant-based and non-bioidentical.

Esterified Estrogens

Esterification is a chemical process that is used to create more complex estrogens. The main esterified estrogens are Estratab and Menest. They are plant-derived but even more removed from the chemical structure of natural estrogens. They are marketed as natural plant-derived hormones that don't have the contaminants of mare's urine, but they are still synthetic.

Synthetic Progesterone-Progestins

Progestins are produced by taking a bioidentical progesterone and altering the molecular structure to make it unique (not occurring in nature) to allow it to be patented. These progestins are also known to be less effective than naturally occurring progesterone.

The most common synthetic progestin is Provera—medroxyprogesterone acetate. It was the main progestin on the market when I was in medical school. It was introduced around 1951 and approved in 1957 as a treatment for amenorrhea (absence of periods) due to hormone imbalance. In the 1970s it became the drug that would try to save ERT. By combining Provera with Premarin, doctors thought they would alleviate the overstimulation of the uterus caused by the "unopposed" estrogens in Premarin.

There were no major studies on Provera until the Women's Health Initiative (WHI) study, which was halted in 2002. The WHI showed that Prempro (combined Premarin and Provera), approved in 1998, increases a woman's risk of breast cancer, heart disease, and stroke and found no difference in endometrial cancer rates between the women who took hormones and those who did not. In other words, Provera does not prevent endometrial cancer, which is the main reason women have been taking it for over thirty years.

Dr. Richard Walker, a New York gynecologist, offers the following comparison between synthetics and bioidentical hormones:

SYNTHETIC HORMONES
- Foreign to the body
- Made from metabolites of horses' urine
- Processed to be "close" in identity to natural hormones
- Long history of unacceptable side effects
- Long-term benefit claims unfounded
- FDA approved
- 200 times more potent than needed

BIOIDENTICAL HORMONES
- Identical to the body
- Made from soy or yam oils
- No history of adverse reactions
- Long-term benefits acknowledged
- FDA approved

The position of the FDA on HRT—as well as that of the American College of Obstetrics and Gynecology and the North American Menopause Society—is that women should go on the lowest effective dose for the shortest possible time and then reassess before continuing the prescription. HRT is now more a choice given to women and not as actively promoted by doctors as it once was. Modern medicine does not, however, take into consideration the natural hormones and make any recommendations regarding their use.

Oral Synthetic Hormone Versus Oral Natural

In summary, drug companies and doctors use synthetic estrogens for three main reasons:

1. Patent and profit.
2. They are more potent than the body's natural estrogen.
3. They are not broken down immediately by the liver when taken by mouth.

To overcome the problem of immediate breakdown of oral natural hormones, two new forms of delivery have become popular—transdermal creams and "micronized" hormones.

Hormone Creams

According to Dr. Richard Walker, current studies show that the best absorption of bioidentical hormones comes from using a cream base. In such a cream, the active ingredients, the hormones, are placed in a cream and applied to the skin. The hormones are absorbed through the skin into the bloodstream. Dr. Walker finds that hormone creams deliver a more consistent and higher concentration of hormones to receptor sites than does the oral route; therefore, the total amount of hormones used is reduced.

The Safety and Effectiveness of Estriol

Safer estrogens may include estriol and bioidentical estrogens, which may be a combination of estrone, estradiol, and estriol. Safer progesterones include natural progesterone. A review paper written in 1998 described the various effects of estriol. The authors reported that in dozens of clinical trials, mostly in Europe, estriol has shown its effectiveness in the treatment of menopausal symptoms including hot flashes, insomnia, vaginal dryness, and frequent urinary tract infections. Studies in Japan confirm estriol's beneficial effects on bone density but results in other studies are equivocal. Estriol is not a hypertensive agent; however, research into its effectiveness in preventing heart disease is incomplete.[38]

Much more funding needs to be direct to researching estriol. We don't know if long-term use will eventually produce endometrial or breast stimulation leading to cancer. Although tested mostly in small clinical trials, estriol has a much less stimulatory effect on the endometrium than estradiol; longer trials are necessary to determine its long term effects on breast and uterus.[39] Some doctors talk about estriol being cancer protective. But it is only recently that animal trials have begun to test this theory.

✄ Who's in Charge of Bioidentical Hormones?

Bioidentical hormones are not promoted by drug companies or by modern medicine in general. They are not patented, and neither have they been thoroughly scientifically researched. But they are very much in the media, mostly because of Suzanne Somers's 2004 book *The Sexy Years*. I've been told that revolutionaries are loved and hated in equal parts by the masses. By taking a very strong stand against synthetic hormones and an equally strong stand for bioidentical hormones, Suzanne made a lot of enemies and a lot of friends. Doctors, mostly male, are outraged that she is "practicing medicine without a license" by telling women to use bioidentical hormones. You can sample their vitriol on Amazon.com in the customer review section on her book. Women, especially those seeking solutions to their menopause symptoms and not willing to risk taking potentially dangerous synthetic hormones, have hailed her book as a lifesaver.

How Much Is Too Much Estrogen?

I don't agree with Suzanne's advice, however, to take bioidentical estrogen and progesterone to achieve premenopausal levels for life. That's not the way the body was designed and we don't know the consequences of such a program. Women who have not touched synthetic hormones get estrogen-dependent cancers because their own bodies produce too much estrogen. We have no way of knowing whether taking bioidentical estrogen might do the same. The fact that there are measurable amounts of xenoestrogens in our environment is also another factor that cannot be forgotten. Taking bioidentical estrogen on top of an unknown amount of xenoestrogens may be dangerous.

Modern medicine, always twenty years behind the times, published a 2004 review of bioidentical hormones in the journal *Menopause*. The authors concluded that "Evidence suggests that, although individualized hormonal products may decrease some symptoms of menopause, it seems they have no proven advantage over conventional hormone therapies and their use is not supported by evidence regarding pharmacokinetics, safety, and efficacy."[40]

If you just read the conclusion of this paper you'd miss the crucial fact that the authors reported that they did not really find enough studies to report on. Their conclusion should state that fact and we should demand more research in this area. In the meantime, the bioidentical hormone market is flourishing through dozens of compounding pharmacies and online pharmacies with people in charge of their own personal experiments!

✤ Bioidentical Hormone Research

Women are pushing the envelope by using bioidentical hormones with or without research. But modern medicine is finally listening to what women want. As reported in April 2004, the University of

Texas Health Center at Tyler studies on bioidentical hormones have begun.[41] At Texas University a Phase I investigational trial was initiated with twenty-nine women using a bioidentical progesterone cream for a twelve-week trial. The results showed:

- No harmful effects of bioidentical progesterone cream.
- Bioidentical progesterone cream relieved menopausal symptoms including hot flashes, sleep disturbances, and depressed mood.
- The cream did not increase clotting factors in the blood.
- The cream had a beneficial effect on levels of certain hormones, including cortisol, a hormone strongly linked to cardiovascular responses to stress in women.

Because the Phase I trial was so successful, Phase II is underway. Doctors were given the green light to study progesterone cream on 100 menopausal women in an ongoing attempt to identify the benefits and any side effects of this treatment that so many women are currently using.

The Texas Study

Dr. Kenna Stephenson, assistant professor of medicine at the University of Texas Health Center and a board-certified family physician, was principal investigator of the Phase I study. "Preliminary findings are exciting for women . . . the beauty of these types of hormones is that they are tailored and individualized to each particular patient depending on her symptoms and her needs," she said. "It's not like the one-size-fits-all of Premarin or Prempro that we know from the women's health initiative (WHI) really didn't have the outcome that we had anticipated."

Because the WHI study showed that women taking Premarin and Prempro had more heart attacks, strokes, and blood clots than women taking the placebo, "we think our findings showing no increase in clotting factors with the progesterone cream is of immense importance," said Dr. Stephenson. "There is a lot of fear about hormones now because of the Women's Health Initiative," she continued. "We want women and their providers to know there are options such as bioidentical hormones that may not confer the same risks as the hormones used in the women's health initiative that also will relieve menopause symptoms." Dr. Stephenson went on to say, "We're interested in bioidentical hormones because we believe it's a safe and smart choice for women at menopause." She recommends that women be tested so the correct bioidentical hormone can be prescribed. "This is the clinical approach that I've used in my direct patient care for a number of years and I have had great success with it," she said.

Micronized Progesterone

I spoke earlier about my experience with prescribing progesterone suppositories for PMS. When taken orally, about 85 percent of natural progesterone is broken down in the liver immediately, rendering it ineffective as a therapeutic drug. You might also say that giving hormones by mouth makes extra work for the liver. The dosages for hormones must therefore be very high to obtain therapeutic effects. To enhance the absorption of progesterone it is now "micronized" and put in an oil base.

An oil base protects the progesterone from destructive stomach acids so that it has a better chance of being absorbed in the intestines and doing its job. Micronization renders the progesterone into very tiny particles that make it better absorbed. Until 1998, micronized progesterone was only available through compounding pharmacies. There are synthetic micronized progesterone products, such as Prometrium, that claim to be natural. However, remember the rule: if it is patented, it has to be synthetic. You can't patent nature. Another reason to avoid Prometrium is that the manufacturer made the bad choice of using peanut oil as a base. Peanut is a major allergen in the population and could have very severe reactions in a certain segment of the population.

Compared to the most common synthetic progesterone (Provera), natural micronized progesterone has very few side effects. Excessive amounts can make you feel sleepy—that's why most women take their dose of progesterone or apply their progesterone cream before bedtime. Unfortunately, not enough doctors have studied natural progesterone, but with the help of their patients they will learn the value of micronized progesterone and progesterone cream and not waste time giving the synthetic forms.

Micronized progesterone from compounding pharmacies does not have to use peanut oil as its base.

Dosage of micronized progesterone is usually 100–200 milligrams per day on a daily basis. In the treatment of PMS, progesterone is taken for the two weeks before the period. The therapeutic amount for micronized progesterone is much higher than for progesterone cream, because there is still a large amount of progesterone broken down by the liver when taken orally.

✖ Hormone Testing

Almost as explosive as the controversy about bioidentical hormones versus synthetic hormones is the method of testing hormone balance. Dr. Stephenson, who was lead investigator of the University of Texas Health Center trial on progesterone cream, suggests that patients should be tested first before going on any hormone treatment. She says, "My patients have been very pleased with this test-and-treat approach, which is an individualized approach to their hormone replacement needs." According to Dr. Stephenson, "Many pharmacies sell saliva test kits, although few U.S. labs know how to read the hormone tests." The Texas Health Center study used ZRT, a lab in Oregon. Dr. Stephenson said, "A doctor would have to get the patient to do a saliva test, send it off and get the results back before prescribing the bioidentical hormone. I believe it's important that the physician and the compounding pharmacist work together as a team in learning what's best for each individual patient."

Saliva Versus Blood Testing

Blood testing to determine levels of hormones is standard in modern medicine. Saliva testing began over twenty years ago. Dr. John R. Lee was one of the first people to become involved with saliva testing. He pioneered the use of progesterone cream for hormone balance and knew that blood testing was an inferior method of measuring ongoing therapy. Elias F. Ilyia, Ph.D., is the director of Diagnos-Techs, Inc., which he established in 1987. It was the first lab in the United States to implement saliva hormone assessment into routine clinical practice. It is the lab I use for my personal hormone testing.

I corresponded with Dr. Ilyia, who said that since 1983, more than 2,500 research papers and articles have been published on the use of saliva as a vehicle for determination of plasma steroid hormone levels. And not just for hormone testing—saliva testing is also used to monitor drug toxicity such as digitalis, celiac disease, liver function, and immunodeficiency. Dr. Ilyia said that progesterone was the first hormone saliva test developed that showed high correlation with clinical symptoms and blood tests. He said that saliva samples are extremely stable and the levels of hormones do not change during shipping. Unlike blood, which is usually drawn in glass tubes, small plastic tubes are sufficient for collecting saliva samples.

Estradiol saliva tests were hampered in the early years by inaccurate tests that did not correlate with plasma estradiol. Present-day saliva tests are extremely accurate and correlate well with clinical symptoms and blood levels. Testosterone saliva tests also correlate well with blood levels. Dr. Ilyia confirmed that estriol, cortisol,

DHEA, and androstenedioine can all be measured with excellent correlation between plasma and saliva levels.

Saliva testing has many advantages:

1. It is noninvasive.
2. It does not require a doctor's presence.
3. It does not require a doctor's fee.
4. It is usually less expensive than blood testing.
5. Samples can be collected in private.
6. The timing of testing can be individualized. For example, melatonin should be checked around 3 A.M.; cortisol should be checked around 7 A.M. In premenopausal women, progesterone should be checked on the twenty-first day of their cycle. Most labs identify the timing of tests on the order form.

Hormone Saliva Testing

David Zava, Ph.D., is the director of ZRT Laboratory, the same lab used in the Texas Health Center trial. He corresponded with me about the difference between blood tests and saliva tests for hormones. He said that the major difference has to do with solubility. Hormones are fat-soluble (dissolve in fat) but blood tests measure water-soluble substances. Hormones measured by blood tests are bound to water-soluble proteins and unavailable to body tissues— they are on their way out of the body.

Dr. Zava said that studies show that about 80 percent of an intravenous (IV) dose of progesterone is taken up mostly by the fatty membranes of red blood cells. Small hormone molecules can travel freely through cells and into saliva ducts. It is these small molecules that can be assayed in saliva. Sex hormones are all very small molecules and all can be tested in saliva. The remaining 20 percent of an IV dose of progesterone is found in the blood and is the amount reflected in blood tests.

Progesterone Creams

Dr. Zava also said that progesterone creams work well because the skin has an underlying layer of fat that allows the fat-loving progesterone to be absorbed. Once in the fat layer, progesterone is absorbed into red blood cell membranes (which have a fat lining), flowing in tiny capillaries traveling through the fatty tissue. Red blood cells carrying progesterone travel to all parts of the body, making their cargo available to target tissues and to saliva. It is this bioavailable progesterone that is measured by saliva and is a better testing fluid than blood.

In fact, Dr. Zava says, when progesterone creams are used by women, and their progesterone levels are tested, there will be a discrepancy; they will appear low. Therefore, researchers will jump to the wrong conclusion and say that progesterone creams are not absorbed. Using progesterone cream will not lead to elevation of blood progesterone but will cause a rise in saliva progesterone levels.

✿ Progesterone Cream and Saliva Testing

According to Dr. Zava, ovulating women have a normal salivary progesterone level of 0.3 to 0.5 nanograms per milliliter (ng/ml). He says that women supplementing with progesterone should aim for that level to restore normal levels of bioavailable progesterone. He says, however, that levels from 0.8 to 1.5 nanograms per milliliter are perfectly safe and benign—especially in women treating PMS, who usually use higher doses of progesterone.

Dr. Zava finds that women who apply 12 to 15 milligrams of progesterone cream daily (compared to 100 to 200 milligrams of micronized progesterone) commonly achieve a salivary progesterone level of 0.5 nanograms per milliliter. Knowing that most progesterone creams contain about 1,000 milligrams of progesterone per 2-ounce jar, dividing 15 into 1,000 give you about 66 days of treatment. For PMS, the dosage may be 30–40 milligrams per day to overcome the "cortisol blockage" on progesterone that is enhanced by severe stress.

Progesterone and Estrogen Balance

It takes two to tango, and that goes doubly for progesterone and estrogen. As I've laid out in several chapters of *Hormonal Balance*, estrogen is often the dominant hormone compared to progesterone. Excess estrogen can dull the sensitivity of estrogen receptors; when they are bombarded with too much estrogen they can partially shut down. When you start taking progesterone cream, however, estrogen sensitivity is restored along with the balance between estrogen and progesterone. Especially if you are already taking estrogen, you can experience more estrogen dominance symptoms such as swollen breasts, headaches, water retention, and weight gain as your estrogen receptors wake up. Estrogen needs to be gradually reduced in such cases. In Dr. Zava's experience, estrogen can be reduced by one-half when progesterone is added and then by half again every two to three months. He finds that most menopausal women do not need to take estrogen once progesterone is restored. Even bioidentical estrogen would therefore be unnecessary, if not unsafe, for long-term use. We have to recognize that the wisdom of the body is to produce high levels of hormones in our reproductive years and to produce lower levels in menopause.

Hormone Balance and Cancer

Dr. Zava had published over fifty studies on hormone balance and cancer. He is convinced that proper hormone balance can prevent many of the sex-linked cancers, especially breast cancer. His 2002 book *What Your Doctor May Not Tell You about Breast Cancer: How Hormone Balance Can Help Save Your Life* (co-written with Dr. John R. Lee and Virginia Hopkins) details his prescription for avoiding cancer. He would agree that postmenopausal women who take synthetic hormones or who have high levels of their own natural estrogen or testosterone are at higher risk for breast cancer than women with lower levels. Dr. Zava repeats his advice that most menopausal and postmenopausal women do not need to take estrogen once progesterone is in balance. And progesterone can be used to balance high levels of natural estrogen in the body.

If You Take Estrogen

Synthetic or natural, because estrogens have been linked with increased risk of endometrial cancer, you still need to have regular checkups and to report any unusual vaginal bleeding to your doctor immediately. The following are tests recommended for people on any form of HRT:

- Annual mammogram (thermograms are preferred, to avoid radiation)
- Annual Pap test and endometrial biopsy
- Annual liver enzyme tests
- Annual hormone testing (preferably saliva)

My Advice on Balancing Your Hormones

If you are still a bit confused about hormones, I don't blame you. I've given you a lot of information to process, the same information I had to process while doing my research. All in all, I really like Dr. Zava's approach to hormone replacement. Here are the steps to take in my recommendations for diet, detox, and nutrients, which I believe are essential before adding hormones.

1. Follow the Menopause Diet that I've outlined in Chapter 11.
2. Detoxify, as outlined in Chapter 7.

3. Take nutrients—vitamins, minerals, essential fatty acids, herbs, and homeopathy—to support your health and to treat mild to moderate symptoms of perimenopause and menopause.
4. If your symptoms continue, have your salivary hormones checked.
5. Take your tests to a doctor and ask for bioidentical hormones for those with low levels.
6. If you can't find a doctor to prescribe for you, seek out reputable online sources endorsed by medical doctors.
7. If your progesterone is one of the low hormones, take that first and evaluate your symptoms by keeping a diary. You may not need estrogen.
8. If you have vaginal dryness, you might ask your doctor for a prescription for estriol cream.
9. Repeat your saliva hormone tests every six months.

It is obvious that bioidentical hormones and saliva testing are both fairly new to medicine. I did not learn about either in medical school and neither did my peers. Most doctors get into this field because they really listen to their patients; they don't want to use harmful synthetic hormones; or they are bothered by their own symptoms or those of their partner. Therefore, you might have to do more of your own research and bring that information to your doctors to light a fire under them. In the Resources section you will find several labs that test for saliva and several compounding pharmacies that make bioidentical hormones.

All and all, it's good news for women. Now we know about xenoestrogens; we know the importance of diet, exercise, and stress reduction; and we are learning about bioidentical hormones. More and more, women have the ability to take control of their health, and to find safer and more effective ways to balance their hormones.

Endnotes

1. Herman-Giddens, M.E.; Kaplowitz, P.B.; Wasserman, R. "Navigating the recent articles on girls' puberty in *Pediatrics*: What do we know and where do we go from here?" *Pediatrics* 113(4) (Apr 2004): 911–17.

2. Frisch, Rose E. *Female Fertility and the Body Fat Connection*. University of Chicago Press, 2001.

3. Forrest, J.D. "Timing of reproductive life stages." *Obstetrics and Gynecology* 82(1) (Jul. 1993): 105–11.

Winter, J.S.D. "Nutrition and the neuroendocrinology of puberty." In *Adolescent Nutrition*, edited by M. Winick (pp. 3–12). John Wiley & Sons, 1982.

4. Frisch, Rose E. *Female Fertility and the Body Fat Connection*. University of Chicago Press, 2001.

5. CDC, National Center for Health Statistics, National Health and Nutrition Examination Survey. Ogden et al. *JAMA* 288 (2002): 1728–32.

6. Corsello, Serafina, M.D. *The Ageless Woman*. Corsello Communications, 1999.

7. Dean, C. "Medical management of premenstrual tension." *Canadian Family Physician Vol 32*: 844–52 (April 1986).

8. Osterweil, N. "Women behaving badly?" *WebMD* (June 18, 2001). *http://content.health.msn.com/content/article/12/1689_51534*

9. Fugh-Berman, A. *Alternative Healing*. Reader's Companion to U.S. Women's History. Houghton Mifflin Web site. Excerpt at *http://college.hmco.com/history/readerscomp/women/html/wh_001200_alternativeh.htm*.

10. Beral, V.; Bull, D.; Doll, R.; et al. Collaborative group on hormone factors in breast cancer. Breast cancer and hormone replacement therapy: collaborative reanalysis of data from 51 epidemiological studies of 52,705 women with breast cancer and 108,411 women without breast cancer. *Lancet*. 1997; 350:1047–59.

11. Lippman, Abby. Bad Medicine: Just Say No. (August 27, 2002) *http://rabble.ca/everyones_a_critic.shtml?x=14959&url=*.

12. Murray, Andy. "Hormone study's end brings Wyeth some relief." *The Eagle-Tribune*, Lawrence, Massachusetts, March 3, 2004. *www.eagletribune. com/news/stories/20040303/BU_002.htm.*

13. PBS Online NewsHour, Hormone Therapy with Margaret Warner interviewing Dr. Marcia Stefanick, July 9, 2002. *www.pbs.org/newshour/bb/health/ july-dec02/hormone_7-9.html.*

14. Bairey, Merz, C.N. "Cholesterol-lowering medication, cholesterol level, and reproductive hormones in women: The Women's Ischemia Syndrome Evaluation (WISE)." *American Journal of Medicine* 113(9) (December 15, 2002): 113(9):723–7.

15. Weed, Susun. *The Menopausal Years.* Ash Tree Publishing, 1992.

16. References for chart:

Ho SM. "Estrogen, progesterone and epithelial ovarian cancer." *Reproductive Biology and Endocrinology.* 2003 Oct 07; 1(1):73.

Martorano, J.T.; Ahlgrimm, M.; Colbert, T. "Differentiating between natural progesterone and synthetic progestins: Clinical implications for premenstrual syndrome and perimenopause management." *Complementary Therapies in Medicine* 24 (1998): 336–39.

Prior, J.C. "Progesterone as a bone-trophic hormone." *Endocrine Review* 11 (1990): 386–98.

Lee, J.R. "Osteoporosis reversal: the role of progesterone." *International Clinical Nutrition Review* 10 (1990): 384–91.

Geary, G.G.; Krause, D.N.; Duckles, S.P. "Estrogen reduces myogenic tone through a nitric oxide-dependent mechanism in rat cerebral arteries." *American Journal of Physiology* 275(1 Pt 2) (July 1998): H292–300.

17. Hoffman, R. "Estrogen dominance syndrome." *Conscious Choice* (Sept. 1999). *www.consciouschoice.com.*

18. Peterson, N. "Havoc in our hormones." *Breast Cancer Action*, no. 36 (June 1996). *www.bcaction.org.*

19. Rajapakse, N.; Silva, E.; Kortenkamp, A. "Combining xenoestrogens at levels below individual no-observed-effect concentrations dramatically enhances steroid hormone action." *Environmental Health Perspectives* 110 (2002): 917–21.

20. Arnold, S.F.; Robinson, M.K.; Notides, A.; Guillete Jr., L.J.; McLachlan, J.A. "A yeast estrogen screen for examining the relative exposures of cells to natural and xenoestrogens." *Environmental Health Perspectives* 104(5) (1996): 544–45.

21. Ulrich, E.M.; Caperell-Grant, A.; Jung, S-H; Hites, R.A.; Bigsby, R.M. "Environmentally relevant xenoestrogen tissue concentrations correlated to biological responses in mice." *Environmental Health Perspectives* 108 (2000): 973–77.

22. Rozati, R.; Reddy, P.P.; Reddanna, P.; Mujtaba, R. "Role of environmental estrogens in the deterioration of male factor fertility." *Fertility and Sterility* 78 (2002): 1187–94.

23. Stapp K. Inter Press Service. New York, May 14, 2004. *www.common dreams.org/headlines04/0515-07.htm*

24. Shaoni Bhattacharya "Viagra could reduce men's fertility." NewScientist. com (January 5, 2004). *www.newscientist.com/news/newsjsp?id=ns99994841*.

25. Gillette, Becky. "Premature Puberty: Is Early Sexual Development the Price of Pollution?" *EMagazine*; November 21, 1997.

26. Ferrie, H. "New perspectives in the war on cancer." *Vitality* (Fall 1999), Toronto, Canada. Visit *www.kospublishing.com* and click on What's New at KOS.

27. *www.cemcor.ubc.ca/articles/misc/perimenopause_ovaries_grand_finale.shtml*. Perimenopause: The Ovary's Frustrating Grand Finale by Dr. Jerilynn C. Prior, MD, FRCPC. Adapted from a Script for Menopause Telehealth Conference Nov., 1998 B.C. Women's Hospital Foundation.

28. Scialli, T.; Fugh-Berman, A. "Perimenopause: an invented 'disease.'" *A Friend Indeed*. May 1, 2003.

29. Prior, J.C. "Perimenopause: The ovary's frustrating grand finale." *B.C. Endocrine Research Foundation* (1:1) (1999). *http://bcendocrineresearch.com/site/*.

30. Dessole, S.; Rubattu, G.; Ambrosini, G.; Gallo, O.; Capobianco, G.; Cherchi, P.L.; Marci, R.; Cosmi, E. "Efficacy of low-dose intravaginal estriol on urogenital aging in postmenopausal women." *Menopause* 11(1) (Jan–Feb 2004): 49–56.

31. Thomas, A.J.; Bunker, V.W.; Sodha, N.; Clayton, B.E. "Ca, Mg and P status of elderly inpatients: Dietary intake, metabolic balance studies and biochemical status." *British Journal of Nutrition* 62 (1989): 211–19.

Bunker, V.W. "Osteoporosis in the elderly." *British Journal of Biomedical Science* 51(3) (1994): 228–40.

32. Cummings, S.R.; Nevitt, M.C.; Browner, W.S.; Stone, K.; Fox, K.M.; Ensrud, K.E.; Cauley, J.; Black, D.; Vogt, T.M. "Risk factors for hip fracture in white women. Study of Osteoporotic Fractures Research Group." *New England Journal of Medicine* 332(12) (March 23, 1995): 767–73.

33. McLean, R.R.; Jacques, P.F.; Selhub, J.; Tucker, K.L.; Samelson, E.J.; Broe, K.E.; Hannan, M.T.; Cupples, L.A.; Kiel, D.P. "Homocysteine as a predictive factor for hip fracture in older persons." *New England Journal of Medicine* 350(20) (May 13, 2004): 2042–49.

34. Halberstam, M.J. "If estrogens retard osteoporosis, are they worth the cancer risk?" *Modern Medicine* 45(9) (1977):15.

35. *www.fda.gov/fdac/features/796_bone.html*. *FDA Consumer Magazine*

September 1996 Issue Pub No. FDA 04-1322C. This article originally appeared in the September 1996 *FDA Consumer* and contains revisions made in August 1997, September 2001, September 2003, and April 2004.

36. Brown, Susan E. *Better Bones, Better Body.* Keats Publishing, 1996.

37. Lieberman, S.J. "A review of the effectiveness of Cimicifuga racemosa (black cohosh) for the symptoms of menopause." *Journal of Women's Health* 7(5) (June 1998): 525–29.

38. Head, K.A. "Estriol: safety and efficacy." *Alternative Medicine Review* 3(2) (April 1998): 101–13.

39. Granberg, S.; Eurenius, K.; Lindgren, R.; Wilhelmsson, L. "The effects of oral estriol on the endometrium in postmenopausal women." *Maturitas* 42(2) (June 25, 2002): 149–56.

Takahashi, K.; Manabe, A.; Okada, M.; Kurioka, H.; Kanasaki, H.; Miyazaki, K. "Efficacy and safety of oral estriol for managing postmenopausal symptoms." *Maturitas* 34(2) (Feb 15, 2000): 169–77.

40. Boothby, L.A.; Doering, P.L.; Kipersztok, S. "Bioidentical hormone therapy: a review." *Menopause* 11(3) (May–Jun 2004): 356–67.

41. Ellis M. "UTHCT starts 2nd study on bioidentical hormones." *Tyler Morning Telegraph*, Tyler, Texas, April 17, 2004. *www.zwire.com/site/news.cfm?newsid=11340303&BRD=1994&PAG=461&dept_id=227937&rfi=6*

Resources

✼ Candida Services

Web site

www.yeastconnection.com

Book

William G. Crook, et al. *The Yeast Connection and Women's Health.* Professional Books/Future Health, 2003.

✼ Compounding Pharmacies

For a national directory: go to *http://dmoz.org/Health/Pharmacy/Pharmacies/Compounding/*

Some of the compounding pharmacies you might contact include:

Hickey Chemists
1645A Jericho Turnpike
New Hyde Park, NY 11040
800-724-5566
E-mail: *info@hickeychemists.com*

Moses Lake Professional Pharmacy
1555 S. Pilgrim Street
Moses Lake, WA 98837
800-476-6505
E-mail: *propharm@atnet.net*

Wellness Health Pharmacy
3401 Independence Drive, Suite 231
Birmingham, AL 35209
800-227-2627

Women's International Pharmacy, Inc.
12012 N. 111th Avenue
Youngtown, AZ 85363
623-214-7700; toll-free 800-279-5708
E-mail: *info@womensinternational.com*

Women's International Pharmacy, Inc.
2 Marsh Court
Madison, WI 53718
608-221-7800; toll-free 800-279-5708
E-mail: *info@womensinternational.com*

IN CANADA:
Victoria Compounding Pharmacy
1089 Fort Street
Victoria, B.C. Canada, V8V 3K5
Toll-free: 1-877-688-5181
E-mail: *wecompound@telus.net*

Saliva Hormone Testing Labs

Diagnos-Techs, Inc.
(Dr. Elias F. Ilyia)
Clinical & Research Laboratory
6620 South 192nd Place, J-104
Kent, WA 98032
800-878-3787

REQUIRES A DOCTOR'S PRESCRIPTION
Great Smokies Diagnostic Laboratory
63 Zillicoa Street
Asheville, NC 28801-1074
800-522-4762 (for doctors)
888-891-3061 (for consumers)

REQUIRES A HEALTH PROFESSIONAL'S PRESCRIPTION
ZRT Laboratory
(Dr. David Zava)
12505 NW Cornell Road
Portland, OR 97229
503-469-0741; fax: 503-469-1305
E-mail: *info@zrtlab.com*
ZRT Hormone Hotline: 503-466-9166. This is a 24-hour taped audio-library with a list of topics on every aspect of hormone balance and testing. Can be purchased directly by the consumer.

Web Sites Featuring Hormonal Health

Centre for Menstrual Cycle and Ovulation Research
Dr. Jerilynn Prior
www.cemcor.ubc.ca

Canadian Women's Health Network
www.cwhn.ca

Index